NICK MITCHELL

YOUR ULTIMATE BODY TRANSFORMATION PLAN

GET INTO THE BEST SHAPE OF YOUR LIFE **IN JUST 12 WEEKS**

For Marcela, without whose love and support this book would not have been possible

Thorsons
An imprint of HarperCollins*Publishers*
1 London Bridge Street
London SE1 9GF

www.harpercollins.co.uk

First published by Thorsons 2016

10 9 8 7 6 5 4 3

A catalogue record of this book is available from the British Library

ISBN 978-0-00-814791-4

Printed and bound in Spain by Graficas Estella

NICK MITCHELL

YOUR ULTIMATE BODY TRANSFORMATION PLAN

GET INTO THE BEST
SHAPE OF YOUR LIFE
IN JUST 12 WEEKS

Thorsons

CONTENTS

NICK MITCHELL

My name is Nick Mitchell and I am the founder of Ultimate Performance – www.upfitness.co.uk, the largest employer of specialist, body composition focused personal trainers in the world. My goal and inspiration in writing this book is to guide you step by step through a total body transformation. I am the only trainer to have taken out-of-shape 'ordinary' men and put them on the cover of all of the leading fitness magazines in the UK, thereby breaking new ground for what is possible for a 'physical transformation'. And let me tell you that you can achieve the results you crave.

But this is no easy ride. There's no sugar-coated advice, no BS here. Ditch the excuses and self-doubt and take the challenge to get into the best shape of your life.

So what are you waiting for....?

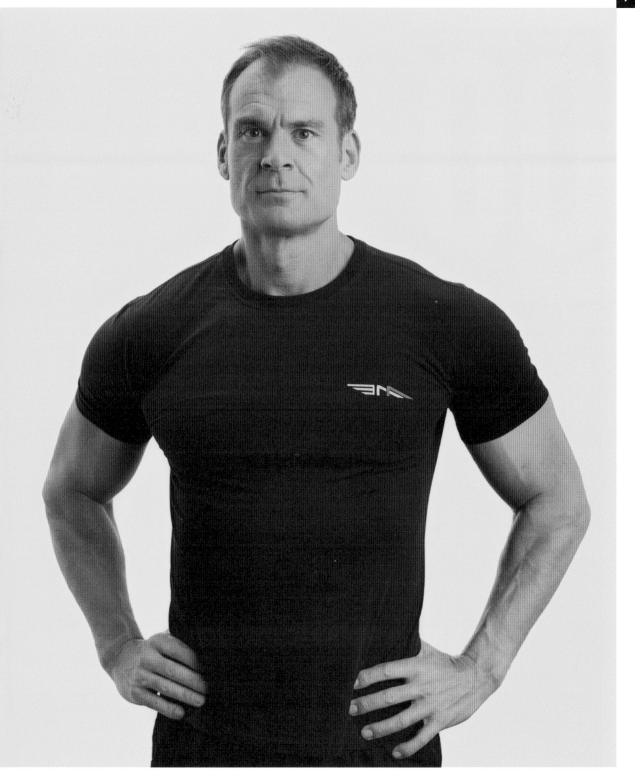

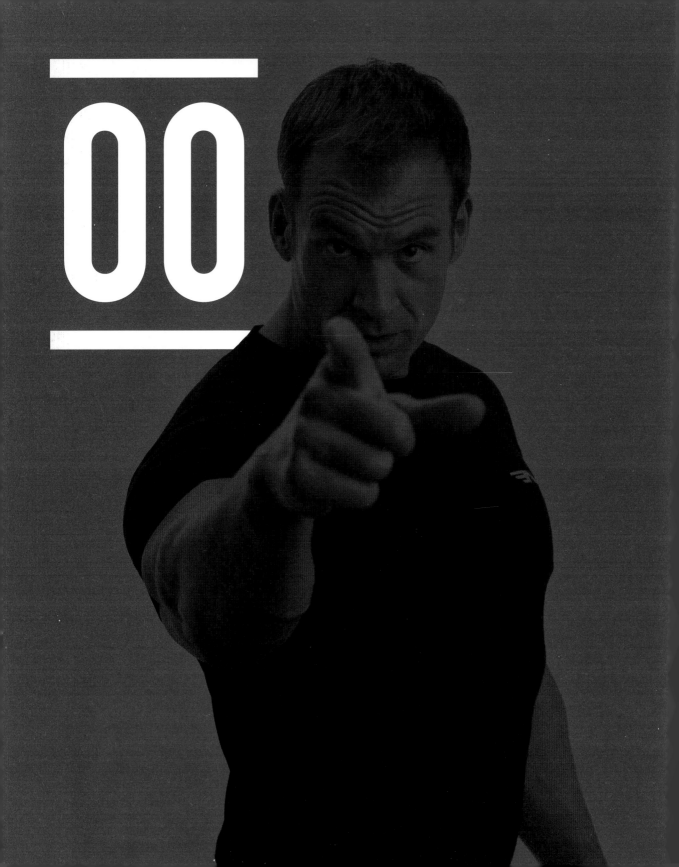

WHERE THE EXCUSES STOP AND THE RESULTS BEGIN

This is a book for those of you who want something a little bit special. It is for the person who has wasted his time trying to improve his body and wants a plan that has worked time after time for thousands of people who live ordinary, non-gym and non-diet-obsessed lives.

I t isn't a book for someone who only ever follows the path of least resistance. If that's you, put this back on the bookshelf now and move on down to an author who tells you what you want to hear, not what you need to hear.

Because now you are in my world.

It's a bit of a strange world to the outsider.

This is a world where we don't foster mediocrity or sell you easy shortcuts.

It is a place where everyone is equal as long as they are prepared to bust their arses with hard work and commitment.

And no matter who you are in the 'real world', when you step into my domain you listen to *me* or you fail.

There is no room and no time for debate and arguments. Save that for the social media wannabes who waste their lives talking and chattering rather than doing.

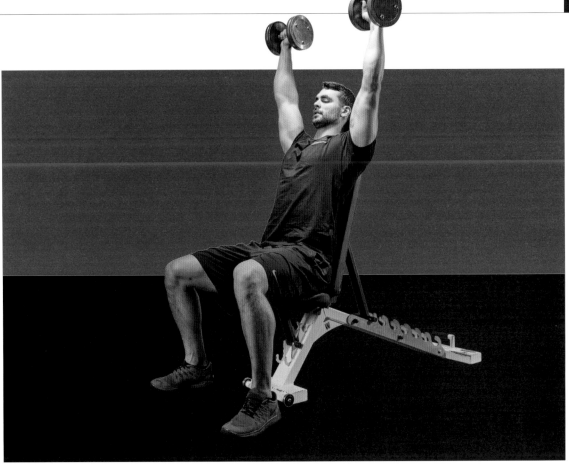

This is the world of hardcore results and the opportunity for those who are willing to take action to finally make a change.

Some of you will go all in and totally transform yourselves.

Others won't be able to muster that level of commitment and will only progress so far. You get out what you put in, and if your ambition is modest then your output will also reflect that. I am not here to judge. I am here to get you the body that your efforts deserve.

I want this book to reflect what I have done with my personal training gyms (www.upfitness.co.uk) which have revolutionised the industry away from 'fitness fluff' into serious and credible results-producing machines. How you employ the machine is up to you; just remember that while the advice contained in these pages is the summation of a huge part of my life's obsession, merely having the knowledge is pretty damn useless unless you have the balls to act.

And not just act for a few days, but to be consistent and relentless when the lazy, procrastinating, excuse-making self that's inside all of us rears his negative ugly head.

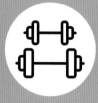

I WILL BE YOUR PERSONAL TRAINER ON THE PAGE

I've been called the world's most successful personal trainer.

I truly don't care about such hyperbolic statements, but what I do care about are two intrinsically linked goals:

1 I always wanted to create a unique business within the personal training industry.

2 I believe that the only way to do that is by being relentless in the pursuit of results over everything else. That means no fluffy towels, zero marketing spend on PR, changing rooms that are a world away from the luxury of our so-called competitors, and every penny and second of time invested in achieving just one goal – *maximum results in minimum time.* My philosophy is solely focused on giving a tangible and valuable return.

MAXIMUM RESULTS IN MINIMUM TIME

Maximum results in minimum time is the essence of this book. If you can grasp that then we have taken the first vital step to you achieving your goals.

I want – no, I *demand* – that you be impatient. If you have no sense of urgency then you will meander, find excuses, and ultimately fail.

What we are going to do in the chapters that follow is set out a blueprint for you to get the body that you want. This is my 'ultimate transformation plan' for men, and it covers everything from what to do in the gym if you're a beginner through to maintenance workouts when you want to cruise; how to eat to maximise muscle gain and how to diet for rapid fat loss; and at the heart of this book is a 12-week training guide that is a first in the world of fitness books in that it gives you control over the parts of your body that you wish to focus upon and improve. You can't reinvent the wheel in this game, but you will find a novel way to make this plan work for you.

As much as it is possible for me to do so I want to act as your own personal trainer.

The beauty of modern technology means that with a bit of extra effort and care we can add so much more than simply delivering this book and leaving you to fend for yourself. In fact, there is a massive danger in that, when it comes to the world of exercise, many of you out there have never been properly exposed to the focused intensity of what a real workout is all about.

Fortunately, or perhaps unfortunately for the pain receptors entwined throughout your muscles, this book is the foundation of your programme, but we can enhance it with all the following benefits:

ONGOING ADVICE WHILE FOLLOWING THE PROGRAMME

The easiest solution of all is that if you have a question about the plan I will personally make myself available to answer you via Twitter at @HeyNickMitchell. All you have to do is put this amazing book cover as your profile pic and then ping your question over.

PROPER EXECUTION OF EXERCISES

We've gone to great lengths to illustrate every single movement in this book so that you know exactly what you're doing in the gym. However, I also accept that there are limitations to two-dimensional photographs. If you want more guidance then you can go to www.UltimateTransformation.Guide or use Shazam to access video downloads of me running through every single exercise contained in this book.

SOCIAL SUPPORT

No man is an island, and while I am very much a proponent of the School of Tough Love, I am much more concerned about getting the job done versus being a hard-ass just for the sake of it. Over at www.UltimateTransformation. Guide there is an exclusive online forum for those of you following the journey and experience of this book. It's a fantastic opportunity to share stories and to inspire, and be inspired by, people just like you.

THE ULTIMATE TRANSFORMATION COMPETITION

If there is one thing that I have learned about what it takes to motivate people to get into shape it is that a clear and defined goal trumps all. We are running a massive competition for those of you who get the best results from the main 12-week programme. All the details are on the website (www.UltimateTransformation. Guide). Trust me when I tell you that throwing yourself into this is the best thing that you can do to make the focused changes you need to transform your body.

WHAT RESULTS CAN YOU EXPECT?

The results that you will achieve are largely a result of three factors:

YOUR PARENTS

I am sorry but I can't control your genetics and you're stuck with the hand that your DNA dealt you. No one can change the shape of your clavicles or length of your muscle bellies. However, this book contains a unique programme that is all about helping you to sculpt your body in an extremely precise fashion. It isn't a generic plan that treats everyone the same.

You can pick and choose the areas that you want to improve upon just as if you were working with me one-to-one in the gym.

TIME

I wish it was possible to create your ideal body in just a few weeks. But results – and one way for you to start thinking of results is as 'positive adaptations to the stimuli that you place your body under' – are always a function of time. Yes, amazing things can happen for some people in even as little as six weeks, but the longer you have the better your results.

This book has a 12-week programme that you can adapt to fit whatever timeframe best suits you. You can follow this book for a year and there is enough variety built in that you won't get bored or stop seeing results. As a little teaser and hopefully a huge inspiration,

here's a before and after photo of one of my most famous transformations. This change, and I promise you there's no digital retouching or even pushing his belly out in the before picture, took Glenn Parker just 15 weeks! You may not want to change as much as Glenn did, but when you look at this your excuses should evaporate.

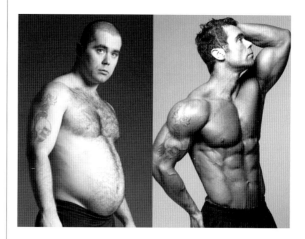

EFFORT

Spot the pattern here? Maximum effort – if channelled intelligently – equals maximum results.

I cannot tell you how much you will change, but I can assure you that if you give it your all you will be astonished by what you can achieve. It is in your hands just as it was in the hands of these men pictured below who followed the 12 Week Body Plan.

MY BODY TRANSFORMATION
BY JOE WARNER

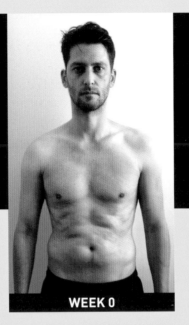

WEEK 0

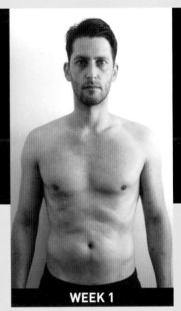

WEEK 1

There are times when I wish I'd never met Nick Mitchell. They don't last long – usually for about a minute every workout when he's pushing me so far out of my comfort zone I think I'm having an out-of-body experience. But that's exactly what you need to do if you want to add the most amount of muscle and lose the most amount of fat in the least amount of time. And there's no one better than Nick at getting incredible results quickly.

I first met Nick about six years ago when I was the deputy editor of the UK *Men's Fitness* magazine. He became a regular contributor, and his knowledge and experience of the body-composition game sparked two thoughts in my mind: was it possible for a 30-year-old to transform his body from marathon runner to cover model? And, if so, how long would it take? Nick's answers – yes, and 12 weeks – came with the caveat that it was only possible if I did absolutely everything he said. I did, and ended up on the cover of the September 2012 issue of *MF*, which was soon followed by the internationally bestselling *12 Week Body Plan*.

We'd proved that it was possible to make astonishing changes to your physique in just three months if you made it your number-one priority and worked your nuts off.

But it turned out that, for me, maintaining my new body was a bigger task than building it in the first place.

BACK TO SQUARE ONE

Fast-forward three years, to April 2015, and I was in the worst shape of my life. There were many reasons why I'd let it slip, but the biggest was leaving my job and setting up my own publishing company,

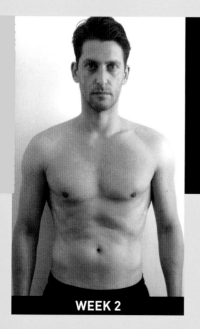

WEEK 2

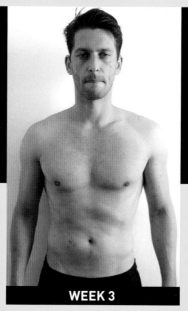

WEEK 3

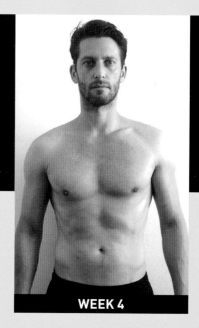

WEEK 4

launching a new magazine app called IronLife. The new business involved a lot of long hours, international travel and huge pressure, as well as having to quickly learn an entirely new skill set, and facing and overcoming new challenges with little experience on a daily basis.

As anyone with a busy job knows, the longer your working day becomes, the harder it is to find the time or motivation to work out. And once your four-times-a-week gym habit morphs into a four-times-a-week pub habit, it's impossible to maintain your current muscle-mass

or body-fat levels, let alone improve them. Eating well becomes harder, too, and soon you're in a vicious circle where you can see your body get into worse and worse shape, and it becomes increasingly hard to get out of the downward spiral.

Before I knew it I was the same weight as I was at the end of my cover-model challenge – around 75kg – but with a body-fat percentage in the mid-20s, rather than in the low single digits. And I looked and felt a decade older than my 33 years.

In short, I was out of shape. In a bad way.

MISSION IMPOSSIBLE

And that's when I got a call from Nick. The next thing I knew I was on a plane to Spain – where Nick has a state-of-the-art gym in Marbella on the Costa del Sol – to be the guinea pig for this book.

To say I was nervous is a bit of an understatement. I don't think I'd ever been more worried about anything I've ever done before. Not only was I in terrible shape and harbouring huge doubts that 12 weeks would be enough time to turn my belly into a six-pack, I was also leaving London at an incredibly critical time for work. The

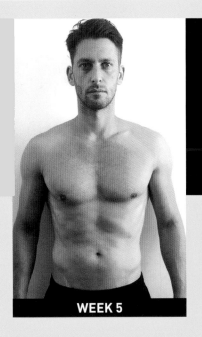

WEEK 5

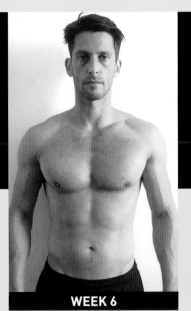

WEEK 6

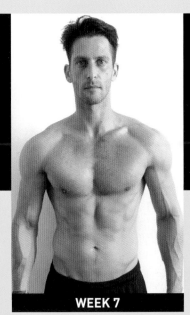

WEEK 7

launch of IronLife had gone so well that we were in the late stages of launching a second magazine, this time a free men's fitness-lifestyle title called *Alpha Man*. I was going to be out of the country and would miss many important editorial and commercial meetings, and all the other essential teamwork behind a new magazine launch.

When I met Nick at the gym the following morning he did little to ease my concerns about whether we were faced with mission impossible – he was unable to stop laughing when I took my top off for our starting week-one photograph. But after sitting me down and talking me through his plan, I remembered why he is one of the best in the business. Yes, he said, I was in a very bad starting position – 'You have cellulite on your stomach. In 30 years I have never seen that on a man' – but I had one key advantage that I didn't have last time: I knew exactly how hard this was going to be.

In that one statement he accurately summed up what lies at the heart of any successful transformation challenge, and that's the right mentality. You need to throw yourself into a challenge like this without hesitation. You need to accept that it's going to be tough and it's going to hurt, and there are going to be times when you want to quit, but you need to want it more than anything else in the world. And seeing the 'Before' picture of my pale and tired face and skinny-fat body, taken moments earlier under the Spanish sun, was all the motivation I needed to make this challenge my number-one priority.

Nick then explained how we were going to crack this challenge. Imagine there are 100 boxes you need to tick to make positive body-composition changes, he said. The more you can tick off at the same time, the faster

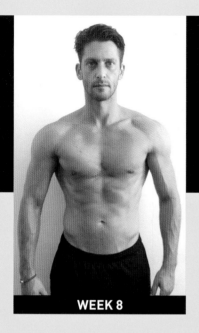

WEEK 8

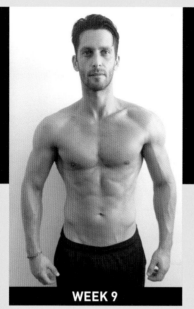

WEEK 9

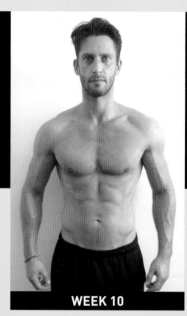

WEEK 10

you'll make progress. Before I arrived in Marbella I was ticking just one of his 100 boxes. It was the first one. The one that requires you to be alive. Now I needed to start ticking as many as possible. His takeaway point was simple: do lots of little things – no matter how seemingly insignificant in isolation – right at the same time, and they quickly accumulate and launch you onto the path of progress.

TICKING THE BOXES

Overnight I dramatically started ticking off his virtual boxes. I started working out – one box – but instead of just going through the motions, under Nick's constant guidance I started training smarter and harder. That's another one. I started thinking about every single rep and focused my mind on how the working muscle felt as I lifted and lowered the weight. One more box. And I swapped thinking about how much I hurt and how much I wanted to stop for focusing on why I was there and what I wanted to achieve. Tick, tick, tick.

I also started eating better. Not just more healthily – I made a total dietary departure from my previous habits of either skipping meals or ordering takeaways, to carefully considering every morsel that entered my mouth. And I made a very conscious effort to improve my chances of falling, and then staying, asleep.

Suddenly I was ticking boxes left, right and centre. And guess what happened? My body started changing shape. And fast. Fat melted away from my mid-section and my muscles started to grow.

My point is that if you want to make a radical change to how you look in your underwear then stop thinking you can out-train

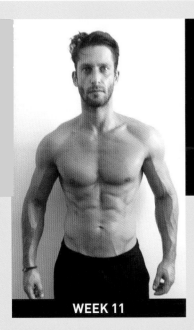

WEEK 11

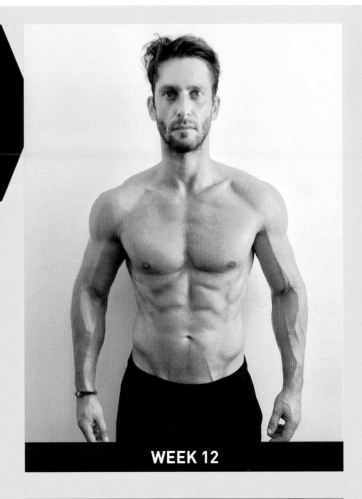

WEEK 12

a bad diet, stop believing that you will get lean by eliminating all dietary fat and stop trying to burn the candle at both ends.

Because the key to a successful transformation is creating a lifestyle that is more than the sum of its parts. The positive effects of doing many little things right don't just add up, they multiply – and the result is even greater gains. Better energy levels, better hormone function, better digestion. Increased fat loss, increased muscle mass, increased positivity. Less stress, fewer cravings, less doubt.

MISSION ACCOMPLISHED?

I don't know yet whether the transformation has been the success Nick and HarperCollins hoped for. I am over the moon with the progress made in such a relatively brief period of time and have never looked or felt fitter, healthier and happier. But whether we've done enough to make this book happen remains to be seen.

I am writing this last paragraph on the flight back to London with the final photoshoot just days away. I guess if you are reading this, then I did it. I transformed my body into one good enough to grace the cover of a book. Now it's your turn.

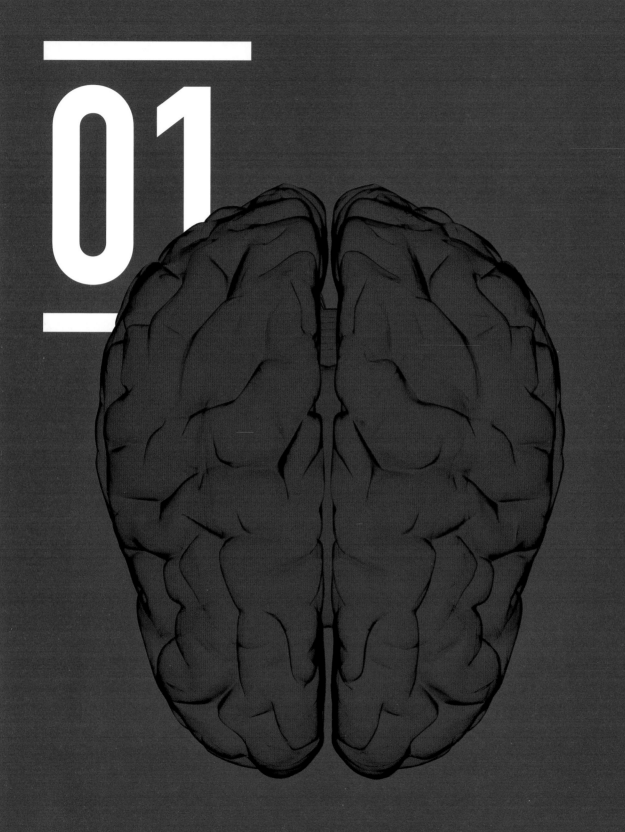

01

GET YOUR HEAD STRAIGHT

Does it strike you as odd that I've chosen to start a book on what many would consider to be an 'exercise and diet guide' with a chapter on mental performance?

f it does seem strange then either you need an attitude adjustment or your brain is already clicked into a higher gear and you can skip this chapter. A rare few will fall into that latter category: congratulations, you're probably successful at most things that you do because you understand the power of *focus*.

DON'T BLAME IT ON YOUR PARENTS

You may think that you are stuck with the body your parents gave you. Your genetics are unchangeable after all. But there is a smart way to create a whole new look to your body. This is what this book is all about.

All forms of exercise are great, but the reason why the programmes in this book are so resistance-training focused is because a correctly executed weight-training regime is far and away the most effective way for you to shape, sculpt and change your body.

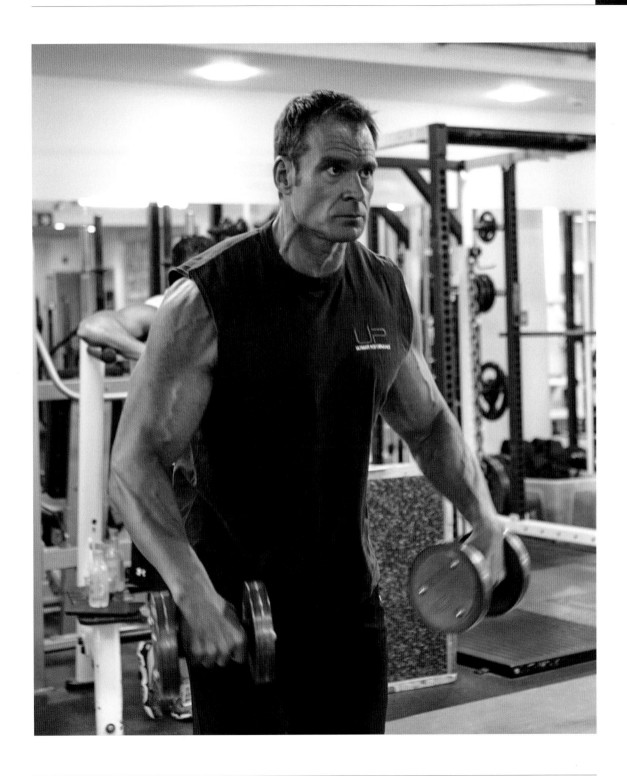

YOU MAY LOOK IN THE MIRROR AND SEE A SHAPELESS LUMP, BUT I SEE A PIECE OF CLAY READY TO BE TRANSFORMED INTO SOMETHING RADICALLY DIFFERENT

You may look in the mirror and see a shapeless lump, but I see a piece of clay ready to be transformed into something radically different. That is one of the key premises in *Your Ultimate Body Transformation Plan*, because it allows *you* to take charge of the areas of your body that you want to improve.

First of all, however, I need to give you a little disclaimer. Slavishly following the guidelines in this book will not give a narrow-shouldered man wider clavicles (collar-bones).

If you have uneven abdominal muscles then they will stay uneven forever. Stumpy, fat legs are always going to be short and, to be frank, a little bit stumpy. Simply put, you cannot change your genetics and beat nature. But what you can do is create an illusion.

Many people think that I have wide shoulders. That isn't true at all, and I'm a bit of a long and lanky beanpole with narrow clavicles. But what I have done is built up my medial (side) deltoid muscles to present an impression of width.

Taking things one step further, by thickening my back muscles and getting a better V-taper I will look broader still. And then tightening the waist and getting leaner is going to further enhance that illusion.

So what you need to do is to take a highly critical look at your own body to see what areas you want to focus on to create the desired 'illusion'. Don't just take photographs; have someone video you from all angles. The reality will be very sobering. But now you have your clay and the sculpture is in your hands.

THE UNIQUE NATURE OF THE WORKOUT PROGRAMMES

There is a trade-off between writing a training programme for the reader of a book, versus writing a programme for someone whom I can see, talk to and assess on a regular basis.

The trade-off is that via the book I get to spread the message of how to really train for results as wide and as cost-effective for you as possible, but at the expense of individualisation. It is a trade-off that I believe is worth it, but it is also an issue that I am acutely aware has never been properly addressed in mainstream fitness publishing.

Until now.

If you want a highly effective broad-based workout that has helped hundreds of thousands of people then all you need to do is go to www.UltimateTransformation.Guide and download for free all of the 12-week workouts from my bestselling first book, *12 Week Body Plan*. The workouts are tough, but highly effective, and will help anyone to improve their body. But I always felt that this programme was simply telling the story of what I did to get this book's cover model, Joe Warner, on the cover of *Men's Fitness* magazine and it left too much out.

What we did to help Joe sculpt his body is unique to Joe and not the exact methodologies that I would have used with anybody else.

This book, which in many ways has taken the premise of *12 Week Body Plan* and improved it in both depth and range, is all about empowering every reader to work on his own unique aesthetic, and to do that I have written what can be best described as a series of exercise routines for you to plug and play at your discretion.

Rather than you following a 12-week programme that is set in stone and requires no planning, you are now going to have to think for yourself a little bit more.

The blueprint is a 12-week base workout where you add specific weekly body-part specialisation routines on top. There are rules that you must adhere to so I implore you to read the workout sections of the book very carefully. For example, 12 weeks of non-stop arms specialisation would actually be detrimental to you building impressive arms and would see you regress.

If you have any doubts then remember that you can ask me any questions at all pertaining to this plan on Twitter (@HeyNickMitchell) as long as you make this book cover your (temporary) profile picture.

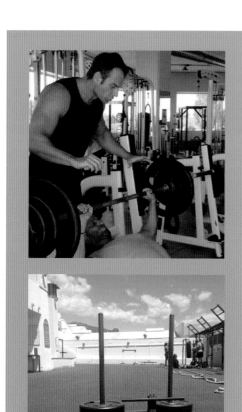

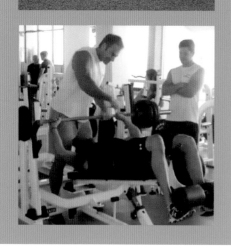

THE SECRET TO MY SUCCESS AS A TRAINER AND THE LESSONS YOU CAN LEARN FROM IT

Do you know why I consistently achieve better results for my clients than any other personal trainer I know?

Why do you think my team at Ultimate Performance (UP) consistently and significantly outperforms the rest of the fitness industry?

The answers to both of these questions may sorely disappoint you. We don't have a secret training programme passed down from Cold War super-scientists. There are no magic legal supplements that will transform you. And even if there were, such things would be available to anybody who could pay for it. The magic illegal supplements (that do work) are off limits and unethical to use unless prescribed as TRT (testosterone replacement therapy) by a medical doctor.

The harsh fact of the matter is that we usually only get our hands on clients for two to three times a week on average. Globe-trotting executives who can afford our fees tend not to stick around in one place and they have highly pressured, stressful careers.

And here's something else that no one in the industry will dare tell you: 80 per cent of people, 80 per cent of the time, pretty much only need the same basic diet (greens, good fats, animal protein, hydration, portion control) to achieve some rather special results.

There is no secret. Except perhaps one.

What has made my professional name is my ability to get inside people's heads. What has made the UP name is our culture that makes the client accountable and gives him nowhere to hide either on the gym floor or when he's home in the kitchen.

I have a unique insight into what works to get results as I oversee the work of over 100 results-obsessed personal trainers. Let me tell you that the smartest and most knowledgeable trainer is by no means the most successful results-producing trainer. In fact very often the more a trainer is obsessed with trying to sound intelligent (a word of advice here: trainers are not scientists, and when they try to sound like one run a mile) the less he focuses on the fundamental basics of ensuring that his client is mentally prepared to do what it takes to achieve his goals.

The single most powerful resource you have to make something happen is your brain. If you can harness your drive, focus and determination then you can achieve so much more than the simple act of transforming your body.

But if you cannot harness your mind's potential then you are doomed to the endless cycle of failure that feeds so much of the fitness and diet industry. I do not want that for you.

THE MYTH OF DISCIPLINE

The best summation that I've ever read on the subject of self-discipline was by the man who taught me more about strength training than anyone else, the world-renowned strength coach Charles Poliquin.

He referred to 'the myth of discipline' and how in the end it all boils down to how badly you want something. Do you really want to have a defined six-pack or do you want those doughnuts? Which one gets you the most excited? It really is as simple and as straightforward as that.

There are various tricks that I am going to teach you in later chapters about how not to succumb to the lure of a doughnut, but we need to go into this process with our eyes wide open. Life is going to get in the way, you are going to stray from the path, but how you react to that and how you reinforce the message needed to achieve your goals is always in your hands.

YOU NEED TO FOLLOW THE RULES OF CHANGE

I TRULY BELIEVE THAT EVERY PERSON WHO IS READING THIS PAGE HOLDS THE KEY TO HIS OWN RADICAL PHYSIQUE TRANSFORMATION.

DEFINE YOUR GOAL/S Decide what you really want to achieve. Write it down. It doesn't matter what this goal is – it could be two inches off your waist or the physique of Schwarzenegger in his prime.

SET A TIMEFRAME ON YOUR GOAL There is a world of difference between thinking 'one day I would like to be ripped' and 'I will be ripped in 12 weeks.' I love the pressure of time-driven goals and embrace them in all aspects of my life, and so should you.

BREAK THAT GOAL DOWN INTO SMALLER TIMEFRAMES If you have a 12-week goal, break it down into bite-sized weekly chunks.

Hitting small milestones on your way to big ones will raise your dopamine levels and keep you focused on the long-term goal. Merely having one longer-term aim can be demoralising when you feel as though your daily efforts haven't made a dent in getting there.

BE REALISTIC I am all for shooting for the stars and am a fully paid-up subscriber to the school of thought that no man, especially myself, should ever hold me back. However, we all need to be realistic. If you only have two hours a week for the gym then cut your goals accordingly.

If you currently carry 35 per cent body fat and would be a welcome new entrant to *The Biggest Loser*, then 12 weeks to cover model is not going to happen.

Dreaming big is part of what makes life fun, but turning dreams into reality is the best thing of all. Make sure that your dreams make physiological and practical sense.

EXERT PRESSURE ON YOURSELF BY ALL MEANS NECESSARY I am a huge fan of using every mental trick in the book to help me achieve my goals. My own personal favourite is to imagine that I am doing a specific task (that is getting hard and I feel like capitulating on) for my children. I visualise their faces in front of me and if I compromise on my efforts in the slightest I will be letting them down.

The nasty cousin of that positive reinforcement is to imagine someone whom you perceive as being an enemy or hater doing better than you. Tell yourself, 'If I don't do this then person X will be more successful than me,' or 'Person Y will be right about me all along.'

My point here is that you should use every driver and motivator possible. Nothing is off limits or should be beyond your imagination!

ASK YOURSELF, 'HOW HARD AM I PREPARED TO GO? WHAT AM I PREPARED TO SACRIFICE?'

Answer this question before you start the programme in this book. Write down your answer. Every time you feel like wavering, return to your original promises to yourself.

HARNESS YOUR FEAR The best

motivator of all is fear. When your back is to the wall you do great things. Do something that scares you – lose a bet, put your photos up on Facebook, or book a photoshoot that you cannot get out of. It doesn't really matter what. All that matters is that you use the fear of failure to sharpen your mind and your actions.

If you embark on this programme with zero accountability for failure then I promise you that you have drastically limited your chances of success even before you have picked up a dumbbell.

WHEN YOU FAIL The only way to

see setbacks is to remind yourself that everyone has them and how you respond right here, right now is what will set you apart from the also-rans and never-made-its.

Embrace temporary failure as the chance to bounce back stronger and harder than ever. Don't allow it to consume you and wallow in it, or you'll kiss goodbye to achieving your goals.

SELF-BELIEF If there is one thing

that I'd love this book to teach you it is the amazing things that you can do once you believe in yourself.

I've lost count of the times that people have told me that until they stepped into one of my gyms they never believed that they could transform their bodies in the way that they have done. That they thought our before and after results were fake or at best done by people who had nothing in their lives but the gym and consuming broccoli and chicken breasts. Once we gave them belief the journey wasn't easy, but it was possible, it all fell into place for them.

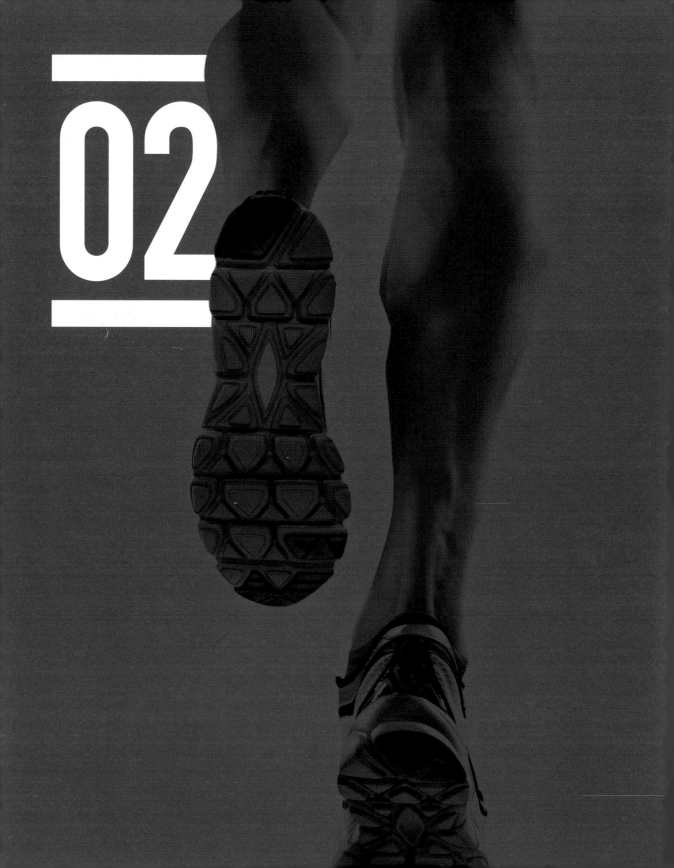

02

LEARNING TO WALK BEFORE YOU CAN RUN

If you find that carrying the groceries from the car to the kitchen is a bit of a workout then it's safe to say that you are a white belt in the world of gym training.

We need you to set off with stabilisers before hitting the mountainous peaks of a real workout.

My advice, if you have been training for less than two years, is to start with the programme in this chapter and follow it for as long as you enjoy it and are making regular strength gains. Typically this will be for anything from three to eight weeks. As a rule of thumb, the more advanced you are as a trainee the more often you need to change your workout.

A quick word on diet. All the training in the world won't change the shape of your body unless you take control of what you eat. While there are such things as advanced peaking strategies that would be inappropriate for someone who is just starting out, the fact of the matter is that you can jump right into your nutritional regime without the need to add a beginner's level 'bridging' period. You can find all the information that you need on how to eat to transform your body in Chapter 6.

MUSCLE-BUILDING AND STRENGTH WORKOUTS

Workouts A and B are to be done on non-consecutive days three times a week.

This means that in any given week you will either do Workout A twice and Workout B once or Workout A once and Workout B twice.

Some of the moves are numbered 1A and 1B, or 2A and 2B. This means that those two exercises form a superset and so are performed in the following way: do all the reps of the first set of the A move, rest for the stated period, then do all the reps of the first set of the B move. You then rest again, if a rest period is stated, then return to the A move and repeat this until all the sets are done, at which point you move on to the next exercise. In Workout A below, 4A and 4B require a different number of sets, so follow 4A and 4B as normal for the first 2 supersets and then, once the second set of 4B is complete, do **just** the remaining set of 4A.

It's really important that you stick exactly to the exercises, sets, reps, tempo (see explanation on page 48) and rest periods listed.

Workout A	Exercise	Sets	Reps	Tempo	Rest	Page
1A	Front squat	3	4–6	5010	120 sec	104
1B	Lying hamstring curl	3	4–6	5010	90 sec	120
2A	Dumbbell bench press	3	6–8	4010	90 sec	96
2B	Shoulder-width chin-up	3	6–8	4010	90 sec	137
3A	Standing barbell shoulder press	3	6–8	4010	90 sec	135
3B	60° hammer curl	3	6–8	4010	90 sec	77
4A	Single-leg calf raise	3	8–10	2110	70 sec	138
4B	Hanging leg raise	2	10–12	2010	60 sec	110

Workout B	Exercise	Sets	Reps	Tempo	Rest	Page
1	Deadlift	4	8, 6, 4, 4*	3210	180 sec	89
2	Rack half-deadlift with shrug	3	6–8	2110	180 sec	106
3A	Decline bench press	3	6–8	3110	90 sec	90
3B	Lean-away pull-up	3	6–8	4010	90 sec	118
4A	EZ-bar reverse curl	2	6–8	2210	0 sec	103
4B	Weighted triceps dip	2	6–8	4010	0 sec	143
4C	Barbell wrist curl	2	10–12	2010	60 sec	81

*The 8,6,4,4 reps refer to the first set being an 8-rep set, the second set you will increase the weight slightly and aim for 6 reps, and for the final two sets the weight will go even heavier and the rep goal drop down to just 4.

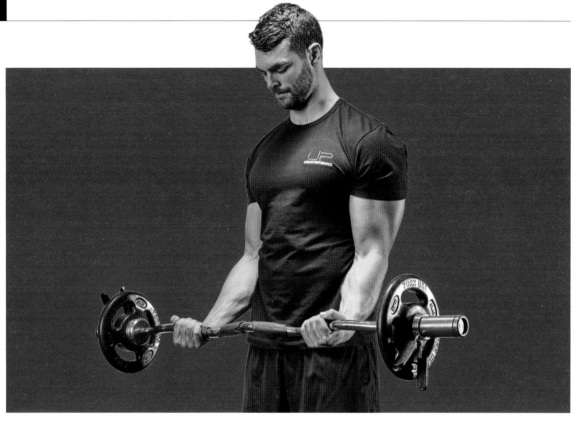

EXTRA WORKOUTS

The weight-training workouts in this chapter are all that you need at the beginner level to stimulate both hypertrophy (muscle growth) and strength gains.

If you are a super-skinny type with the overriding goal of beefing up your frame then these workouts should be all the vigorous exercise that you do until you progress to a more advanced stage. For you, the rule of thumb should be to focus on recovery and relaxation when not in the gym.

Most of you reading this will not fall into that camp and you will have some timber to shift from your middle. Sadly for you, taking it easy isn't an option!

Lesson number one, however, is not about exercise, but instead should be all about your diet. Abs are very rarely made in the gym. They are made by controlling yourself in the kitchen. Following the right diet for a sustained period of time is paramount to achieving your goals, and we delve into this in depth in Chapter 6.

However, many of you will benefit from additional cardiovascular-oriented training sessions. Go to Chapter 4 to read all about the best ways to incorporate cardio training into your transformation programme.

HOW TO LIVE YOUR LIFE (FOR 12 WEEKS): LIFESTYLE RULES FOR MAXIMUM RESULTS IN MINIMUM TIME

Some people say that diet is 80 per cent of the battle for a successful body transformation. Others say that training is 50 per cent. And you will get the wise old souls who say that it's 33 per cent training, 33 per cent diet, 33 per cent rest, and 1 per cent luck! All of them are right. In certain cases.

The blunt truth is that it is impossible to categorically define the exact importance of each factor. It will always be slightly different because we all have different genetics, different starting points and different goals. There are key rules, however, that you need to adhere to if you want a superlative result.

CONSISTENCY IS KING

One enormous problem that I see all the time, and that you may well have suffered from personally, is the lack of appreciation that most aspiring muscle-builders have for the importance of consistency.

The importance of consistency is what makes bodybuilding one of the hardest 'sports' imaginable, because you are effectively working towards your goal 24 hours a day, and the chances are that if you are not doing something positive then you are doing something negative. We all need to remember that the body doesn't stay in some sort of halfway house where it just stays the same: we are either anabolic (building up) or we are catabolic (breaking down). There

is no middle ground here so the inconsistent trainee always becomes the unsuccessful trainee. It is imperative that you are consistent with:

● Your diet. Forget all of this intermittent fasting craze. It is categorically not the best way to build muscle as fast as possible. Some of you will need to find ways to get in as many calories as possible so every opportunity to eat must be taken; others will need to watch every morsel that enters their mouths.

When wanting to add muscle most typical ectomorphs do not consume enough food, so forget about all that you read on the internet about long breaks in between meals to aid protein synthesis and instead focus on getting enough calories and the right macronutrients in and be consistent with whatever feeding schedule is most appropriate for you. The chances are that it will mean consuming calories every few hours and never ever skipping a meal. This will arguably be the most challenging aspect of your transformation process.

● Your training. Going to the gym consistently for two weeks and then skipping five days – a typical routine for the majority of gym-goers – will get you nowhere fast. Yes, you will improve a little bit for a little while, but very soon even the mediocre gains will come crashing to a halt and you will become dispirited, demotivated, and quit. Your body does not want to be lean and muscular and you must fight it tooth and claw to positively adapt to the training stress that you put it under.

 ## PRIORITISE YOURSELF

Radically changing your physique is one of the hardest challenges you will ever undertake. Hopefully you've got the message by now that it takes round-the-clock attention and dedication, and this means that at certain times you are going to have to be selfish. For the next 12 weeks you need to make a deal with yourself and all those around you that for this short period of time you're going to prioritise yourself.

This doesn't mean that you can say, 'Nick Mitchell says it's OK for me to be a selfish bastard or his book won't work.' Far from it, because in order to grow you also want to minimise your headaches!

What I am telling you is that your training, your 'strange' diet and your rest come first. Late night out with the boys? Skip it. Long weekend in the countryside with the wife? Skip it. Running the London Marathon? Skip it. You get the picture. It's only 12 weeks of your life, then you can cruise along, keep your gains, and put your foot down on the gas again when you think the time is right to improve even more.

 ## MAKE MUSCLE YOUR NUMBER-ONE PRIORITY

Unless you're a mutant super-freak the bad news is that your body doesn't want to add muscle. It will fight you every step of the way. And as for adding muscle quickly, just forget about it. Muscle is metabolically inefficient, meaning it uses up too much fuel (which is a positive if we want to look good, but not ideal for the feast-or-famine scenarios our DNA wants us to be prepared for) so your body will look for every opportunity possible to not add muscle. This goes double for those of you who are ectomorphs and naturally slim.

As a result we need to revert to an old bodybuilding maxim of 'not wasting calories'. Don't run when you can walk. Don't walk when you can stand. Don't stand when you can sit. Don't sit when you can lie down. Of course you don't need to take these words literally but it does mean that for the 12-week period of this programme I don't want you playing football, jogging in the park or dancing until 4 a.m. You grow when you rest. Bear that in mind at all times.

And just a quick note for those of you who might be worrying about this advice and the impact on your cardiovascular health. Go through one of the prescribed weights workouts, sticking to the right tempo (see page 48), load and rest intervals, and then tell me that your cardiovascular system 'needs' you to go running!

Please note that the above advice refers to those of you seeking to add maximum muscle, not a 'body recomposition' where fat loss is a critical goal.

📅 PLAN AHEAD

The beauty of the Ultimate Transformation Plan workouts is that all the training is laid out for you. It is easy to follow and you don't need to think about it too hard. The same principle needs to apply to the rest of your life, and whereas it would be impossible to lay out a life plan for you as every reader will have a different job, home environment, and ability to commit, you can and should take control and plan everything out for yourself.

This doesn't mean that you need to sit down and map out everything that you're going to do for the next 84 days. But it does mean that living each day on the fly just won't cut it.

Your gym time needs to be set into your schedule, your bedtime needs to be regular, your eating time needs organising. Above all else your food for the day needs preparing before you leave the house. Popping out for a quick sandwich at lunchtime is guaranteeing you fail this programme. Buy some Tupperware, plan ahead and cook your meals the night before, and make life simple and easy for yourself. Nothing in the plan is difficult – except maybe the training routines! – but it will be mildly inconvenient until you get into the habit of planning ahead. Then it should be as easy as falling off a log and your progress could be spectacular.

MINIMISE STRESS

One of the personality traits that typifies a significant percentage of 'easy gainers' – yes, there are people out there who can add ridiculous amounts of muscle drug-free in a very short space of time – is that they are very laid-back. Conversely, think about people you know who are highly strung: the chances are that they are wiry and lean with very little fat and muscle bulk.

One of the reasons for this is that when we are stressed out and worrying (usually for no good reason) our adrenal glands are working overtime producing the fight or flight stress hormone cortisol.

Cortisol is not the demon hormone that some have made it out to be. We need it to mobilise fat as energy, and without it you literally wouldn't get out of bed in the morning.

However, while acute levels of cortisol have a purpose (running away from something dangerous or getting ready for a hard gym workout), chronic cortisol secretion caused by 'over-stressing' can have a very negative effect in the long run by both lowering our peak cortisol output, meaning that we have lower energy levels and fatigue more easily, and reducing testosterone levels.

Testosterone, as you may know, is the key androgenic hormone that helps us to build muscle tissue and recover from intense training sessions, and is something that we want to maximise as much as possible.

A good way for you to contextualise this is to think about your own sex drive when you're relaxed and on holiday versus a time of extended stress. When you're chilled out and not worrying, your sexual appetite – therefore testosterone level – is much higher than when you're worried and your cortisol is through the roof.

What all this means for you is that in order to optimise your muscle-building efforts you must exercise a disciplined mind and make every effort to only worry about the things that really deserve your concern. Your family, your health and your job are all important. The person who annoys you on the commute to work, the fact that your wife makes you do the washing up, or that bloke off the TV, are all just bothersome things and not worthy of any stress at all. And when you're struggling try this little trick of mine: Ask yourself whether it will bother you five years from now. The answer is almost always a resounding no.

SLEEP IS A NECESSITY, NOT A LUXURY

Sleep is so critical to your progress that it deserves a chapter all to itself. To be very clear, if you do not prioritise a restful night's sleep you will not make optimal progress. I don't care how hard you train and how smart you diet; without the right amount of quality sleep you will never make significant changes to your body.

For those of you who say that you don't have time to get the recommended eight hours of sleep a night, welcome to my world. I am forced to do what Arnold Schwarzenegger says and get six hours by 'sleeping faster', but I am no longer prioritising my body composition. For the purposes of your own 12-week transformation you should insist that you do everything possible to get as much sleep as you need.

How do you define how much sleep you need? You should wake up feeling refreshed without the need for an alarm clock. That's probably something that very few of you ever achieve. It doesn't have to be eight hours, though – for some it will be more, and others can function optimally on much less.

Whatever your own sleep sweet-spot you must never forget that it is one of the key non-negotiables to optimal health, hormones, performance, and physical potential. In very simple terms, not getting enough sleep plays havoc with:

- **TESTOSTERONE PRODUCTION:** Go a few nights on 60 per cent of the sleep you need and see what happens to your sex drive. A teenager or young man in his 20s won't feel this, but wait until the 30s and 40s hit.
- **INSULIN AND CORTISOL:** Your tired mind – never forget how significant the brain is in these things – and body need boosts in cortisol to get them going and they also become more insulin resistant (meaning it is much more likely to store glucose in the fat cells). What sort of foods do you reach for when you are sleep deprived? The worst kinds always – forget meat and veg and think croissants and candy. You do this for a hormonal reason and it will send you into a negative spiral of worse food, lower 'real' energy, mental fog and fat accumulation.
- **GROWTH HORMONE (HGH) PRODUCTION:** We release a lot of our HGH during certain cycles of sleep. Miss these cycles out and you can't play catch-up.

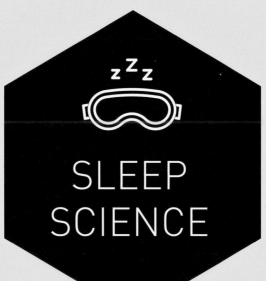

SLEEP SCIENCE

Sleep is much more complicated than you may think, with four distinct stages. There are three non-rapid eye movement stages and the rapid eye movement state, which is associated with dreaming.

In each phase biochemistry is altered within the body to promote memory retention and increase hormonal production.

The first two phases of sleep are the transition period from a state of being awake to that of reduced body temperature and slower brain waves.

The third phase – known as slow-wave sleep – is that of hormonal production and receptor sensitivity regulators. It is critical for body composition change because during this phase your body resets insulin sensitivity and promotes growth hormone production. If you wake up between 1 a.m. and 3 a.m. in the morning after falling asleep at 10 p.m. the chances are that this crucial phase of sleep is disturbed.

Your liver is responsible for much of the hormonal balance, so if the liver is unable to fully process toxins this balance is disturbed and the effect will be a lack of urinary control and a need to use the bathroom during the night. The problem with disturbing slow-wave sleep is that in this phase the switch is reset to prevent the onset of diabetes or cancer growth, so it is vital not only for composition change but also for much more important health factors.

The final phase is REM sleep, which is responsible, among other things, for establishing motor unit function and memory retention.

Therefore sleep can be a complicated process, and for many people it sadly isn't as simple as climbing into bed and hoping for the best. Most of you reading this will not have optimal sleeping patterns, but there are many things that we can do to improve that.

01 Keep regular hours: go to bed at the same time every night and dispel this notion that you can play 'catch-up' at weekends.

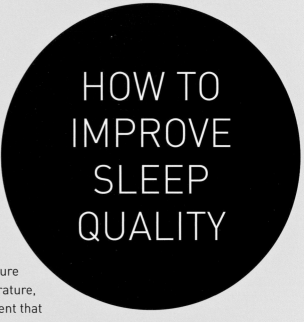

HOW TO IMPROVE SLEEP QUALITY

02 Sleep in a cool room: by decreasing body temperature and regulating room temperature, you can create an environment that will sustain REM sleep.

03 Make your bedroom a Batcave: REM sleep can easily be affected by noise pollution and light interference, so make your bedroom as dark and as quiet as possible. Go as far as switching off electrical devices that have standby lights on. Light interference can easily create a sensory marker in the brain that disturbs REM sleep, therefore it is vital to establish the best sleep environment. Even the slightest light contact with the skin will reduce the quality of REM sleep, so the darker the bedroom the more likely you are to gain quality REM sleep. I know this sounds a bit over the top but the changes will be worth it.

04 Take magnesium. This mineral is vital in aiding cortisol management and therefore assists slow-wave sleep by resetting insulin sensitivity. Magnesium is also a catalyst in re-establishing adrenal health through the cortisol/insulin connection.

05 Take Californian poppy extract. This is a great adaptogenic herb (see page 247) that relaxes brain waves into slow-wave sleep. It also acts as a liver detoxifier and has a secondary pathway in slowly aiding the removal of toxins that affect the sleep cycle.

06 Eat better. Our diets have a significant impact upon the sleep cycle. Foods that are high in carbohydrates may increase serotonin production (the neurotransmitter responsible for a calm, happy and relaxed state of mind), but the downside is that once blood-sugar levels decline the body will go into a natural hunger mode and it is possible that you may wake up as a natural reaction to low blood sugar. Foods that are high in essential fats will aid in establishing a constant blood glucose level, which is beneficial because the body will be able to go into a fasting state while slow-release energy is being made available for metabolic function. Therefore one option to try is to stay away from carbohydrate-rich meals at least two hours before bed and instead have a meal rich in essential fatty acids. You must experiment to find out which approach works best for you as very often, especially in individuals dieting on lower-carbohydrate diets, carbs prior to bedtime can significantly improve sleep quality.

07 If you are waking up after two to four hours of sleep you may benefit from a protocol that will assist your liver's ability to detoxify. Increase fibre intake and consider a morning and evening addition of a high-quality fibre supplement.

- Glucuronic acid, a carboxylic acid with a structure similar to glucose, is vital in unbinding phase-two detoxified substances for removal from the gastrointestinal (GI) tract. Take two calcium d-glucarate capsules three times daily for 16 days.
- Use an oestrogen control protocol (see Chapter 8) for 16 days.
- As an ongoing liver support formula, mix one to three tablespoons of a good-quality greens powder (a concentrated version of several fruits, vegetables and herbs that is taken as a supplement) with 1.5l of water and consume daily. Maintaining pH levels will aid not only GI detoxification but also positively influence proper cortisol management.

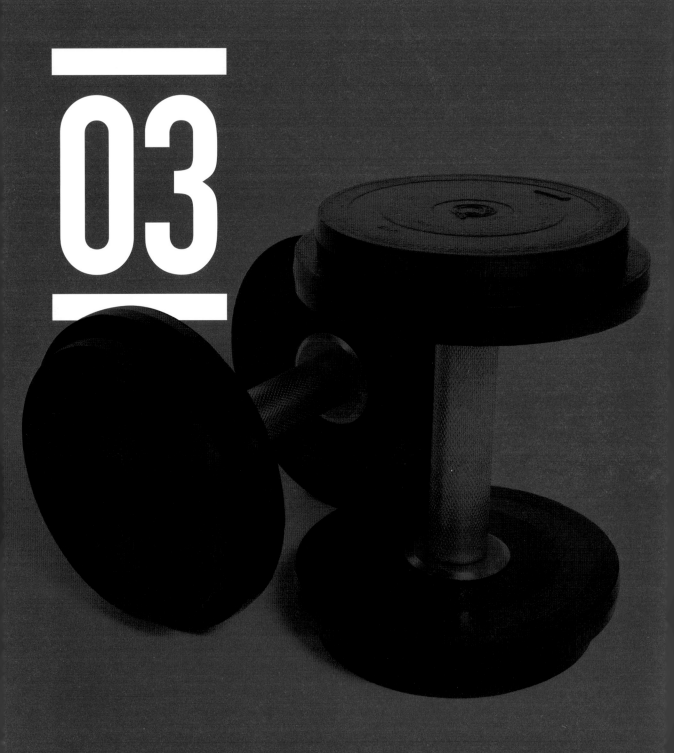

03

EXERCISE FUNDAMENTALS

'To progress in the gym you must do today what you could not do yesterday.' If only the hordes of gym-goers worldwide could understand this concept then gym results would be magnified tenfold.

Only by forcing your body to a place that it doesn't want to go will it make a positive adaptation, in this case by getting stronger, fitter and laying down new muscle tissue.

I want to set out some rules for you to live by when you go to the gym. If these concepts are new to you then please read through them before every single workout until they are ingrained in your brain. They really are that important.

HOW TO LIFT WEIGHTS

I'd hazard a guess that the average gym-goer should be considered a failure when it comes to achieving their weight-training goals. This would be for multi-factorial reasons, but one critical missing component is that very few people know how to properly lift weights. If you think that effective weight training is all about lifting a weight up and putting a weight down then you need to completely rethink your approach.

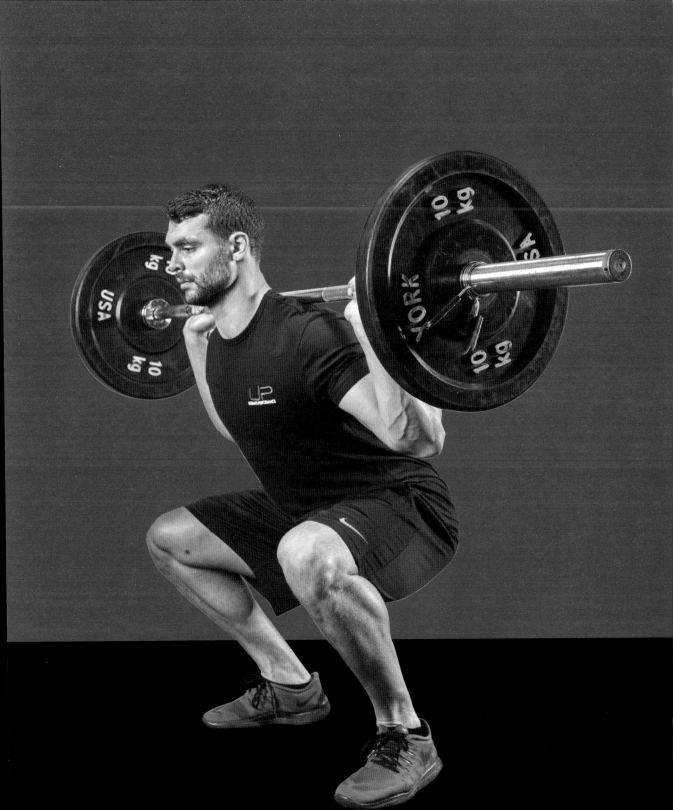

Before we get into what that new approach should be I want you to ask yourself a question. What are you trying to achieve when you are resistance training?

If your answer is 'to show off to hot chicks in the gym' then you and I have reached a philosophical crossroads and we need to part ways. If your answer is the slightly more complicated 'to use progressive overload and improve by lifting more weight or doing more repetitions at every session' then you do have half the answer, but you are also running the risk of falling into the trap of chasing performance at the expense of stimulation, and often safety.

The correct answer if you want to go from gym zero to gym hero is that your resistance-training focus should be all about placing maximum stress on your muscle fibres in order to stimulate the most powerful adaptive hypertrophy response. Or in plain English – muscle growth!

Does this mean that you shouldn't strive to outperform your last workout? Absolutely not. The principle of progressive overload holds very true and you should always aim to 'do more than before'. But the old adage that your muscles do not know the number of the weight that you are lifting is also very true. Actual weight lifted is irrelevant for your muscle-building progress; it is all about the stress imposed on the muscle fibres. Of course, part of that stress is caused by the weights that you lift, but maintaining tension on the muscle you are training is of unrivalled importance. Lifting things up and putting things down does not cut it if you want the best results.

The one single trait that all successful trainees have is the skill to focus on not simply moving the weight from point A to point B, but instead to emphasise the ultra-important necessity of flexing the muscle against the given resistance to achieve the hardest possible muscular contraction.

When executed properly a biceps curl isn't simply flexing the elbow to get the wrist to the front shoulder. If that's the way you currently curl, next time you do it decrease the weight by 75 per cent, close your eyes, and simply focus on contracting your biceps as hard as possible.

If you are attempting to elicit the strongest possible stimulation then you should always remember that the weight is a mere tool in your hands, and it is how you contract your muscles against that weight that will get you results. To really achieve the best results for all your hard work in the gym you need to learn how to milk every rep of every set for all it's worth.

If you lack the neurological connection to a muscle, more commonly known as the mind–muscle connection, do some unilateral (single-limbed) work and place your free hand on the working muscle. This can really help you feel the muscle contract. By way of example, the back muscles are among the hardest to feel working, so if you really struggle here ask a training partner to touch your back in the places that it should be working.

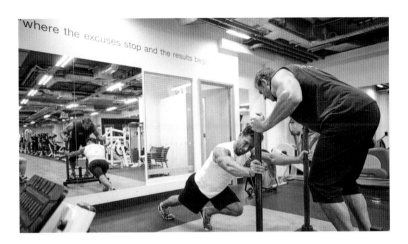

CHANT YOURSELF A MANTRA. IT IS ALL TOO EASY TO GET CAUGHT UP IN THE NUMBERS

While I have just emphasised the need to flex your muscle against the weight rather than simply heave and hoist it up, it is an unarguable fact that when you can go from six strict-form chin-ups with your bodyweight to six equally strict chin-ups with 25kg tied around your waist, your biceps and upper back will be larger and thicker.

So you do need to chase the weight and the repetitions, all while focusing on the right way of lifting.

I could easily devote half of this book to the art of correct contractions for muscle building – it would need a snappier title than that – but we don't need to make it too complicated. There are two very simple mechanisms to drill into your head when performing almost every exercise in this book, and if you do have any doubts after looking at the step-by-step guides (see page 74) then pop over to www.UltimateTransformation. Guide or Shazam the images to watch the relevant exercise demo videos.

On every single repetition of every single set I want you to tell yourself to 'stretch and squeeze'. As you contract the working muscle what you are actually doing is shortening it. Draw your arms across your chest and you shorten your pectorals. Flex the muscle in your front thigh (quadriceps) and again you shorten that muscle. Giving yourself the mental cue to 'shorten' is a bit flat and limp, so instead you should tell yourself to forcefully 'squeeze'. Top professional bodybuilder Ben Pakulski uses the line 'squeeze it like it owes you money'. You can never squeeze a muscle too hard.

We squeeze or shorten the muscle as we flex with what is referred to as a positive or concentric contraction, best envisaged as raising the weight. We stretch or lengthen the muscle as we lower the weight in what is referred to as a negative or eccentric contraction (see page 263).

It is imperative that you fully exploit the benefits of both types of muscular contraction, which means a forceful squeeze for the positive rep and a controlled and measured, never ballistic (bouncing), stretch as you lower the weight to the bottom of the given movement's range of motion, or ROM.

WARMING UP, PROPER WEIGHT SELECTION AND TEMPO

Running straight from the changing room into your first set without warming up isn't only dangerous, it's also stupid. A proper warm-up not only prepares your muscles for what lies ahead – helping prevent an unnecessary injury – it also fires up your central nervous system (CNS), which means your muscles will contract quicker, making you stronger, when the real workout begins.

But if you thought that the best way to warm up was five or ten minutes on the treadmill, it's time to think again. How can a gentle jog prime your muscles for a hard weights session, especially if you're training your upper body? Here's what you need to do.

WARM UP

The most effective way to warm up your muscles is to perform progressively heavier versions of the moves you are going to be doing. So you'll start with a few reps at an easy weight, then gradually increase the weight, while keeping the reps low as you want to minimise fatigue, until you work up to your target work-set weight. Here's the formula you should stick to to ensure you select the right weights for each warm-up set.

Say the first move of the workout is squats and your target work-set weight is 100kg for 10 reps.

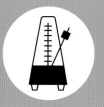

TEMPO EXPLAINED

The use of correct lifting tempo – or the speed at which you lift and lower a weight – comes into play here because the proper application of stretching and squeezing on each repetition is what places tension on the muscles. Later on in the book when we get to the actual workout programmes you will find that every single exercise has a prescribed tempo. Don't get lazy and mess around with the tempo times. They are there for a reason, and the closer you adhere to them the better your results.

Tempo is detailed by a four-digit code, such as 2010. The first number is the time in seconds that the weight is lowered; the next number is the time in seconds that the move is held at the bottom position; the third number is the time in seconds that the weight is lifted; and the final digit is the time in seconds that the weight is held at the top of the move.

WARM-UP SETS

Warm-up set one:
8 reps at 30 per cent (33kg),
minimal rest.

Warm-up set two:
5 reps at 50 per cent,
30–60 seconds rest.

Warm-up set three:
3 reps at 70 per cent,
45–75 seconds rest.

Warm-up set four:
2 reps at 85 per cent,
60–75 seconds rest.

Warm-up set five:
1 reps at 95 per cent,
60–75 seconds rest

Start first work set.

You only need to do this for the first two moves of your workout. For all subsequent moves for the same or similar body parts select a weight that is about two-thirds that of your work-set rep and perform 4–6 reps to get the motor pattern right, but if you are moving to a totally cold body part do begin this warm-up sequence again – you'll not just be safer from injuries, you'll also be stronger. If chin-ups, pull-ups or dips are in the first two moves, then use a resistance machine to warm up instead.

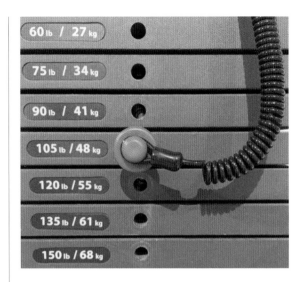

ACTIVATION

Explosive movements before your initial work sets can further activate your central nervous system (CNS) to elicit greater reaction and force from your muscles. We don't need to make this complicated: simply think of the exercises you have coming up and try to mimic them with explosive movements. Before pushing exercises you can hurl a medicine ball at the ground as hard as possible, do a couple of clapping press-ups, or even unleash a left and right hook on a heavy bag. For lower body exercises, a hard kick (with each leg, of course) on the heavy bag will do the trick, as will two to four jump squats. The key with nervous system activation is to move as quickly as Joe Warner when it's time to pay the bar bill!

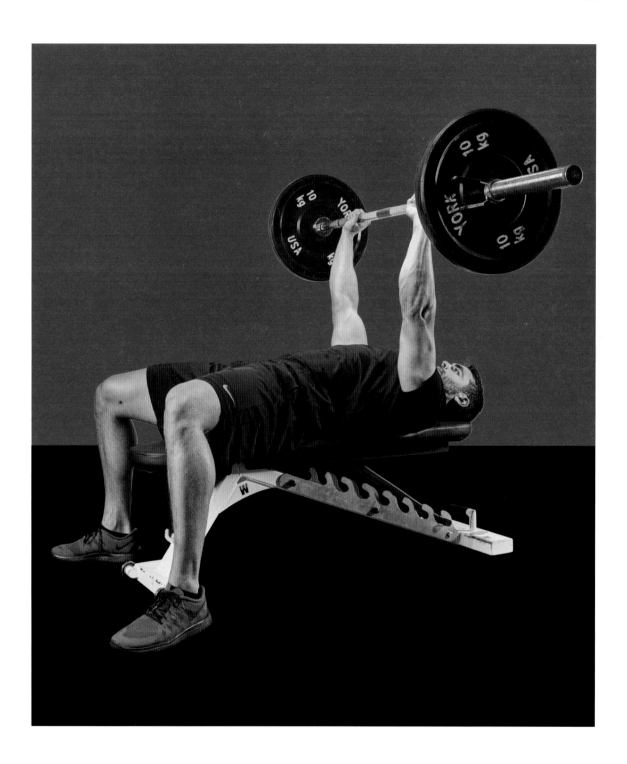

THE RIGHT WEIGHT SELECTION

Selecting the appropriate weight for a set is of paramount importance. From time to time I still see personal trainers who can't seem to select the optimal load for their clients, and guess what, these are the clients who never quite achieve stellar results. Typically, the mistake is that the weight is too light and the set is too easy, but walk into any bodybuilding gym and very often you'll observe the opposite mistake. They should take my advice: train with 'the brain of a woman and the heart of a man'.

For those of you who are offended by that please tuck your vest back into your nappy and understand that all I mean is that most women would benefit from being a bit more aggressive in the gym, and most men would benefit from checking their egos and thinking about what load will allow for the most stimulation of their muscles and not their alleged gym reputation. If you think I am speaking directly about you with this message, then it's time to change things up. Your results will increase exponentially if you can make better decisions about which weight to use.

Weight selection determines almost everything you do in a set.

The main variables in a set are repetitions, tempo, correct lifting form (this shouldn't be a variable, it should be perfect, but we know form can suffer as a set gets harder), time under tension (TUT) and load, so what is going to happen if you pick the incorrect weight?

Everything else gets thrown out of the window, that's what. And then the specific effect that you are seeking from that particular set will be lost. This is one of the most fundamental aspects of your training that you simply can't afford to get wrong. While I can give you an awesome, spleen-busting, results-producing training programme on paper, if you don't select the right weight for yourself then it could be a total waste of time.

I have long held the belief that training with heart and no brains trumps training with brains and no heart, and nowhere is this more apparent than in the interpretation of a written programme.

There is no point in being a stickler for TUT, reps, rest intervals and tempo if you pick a weight that doesn't challenge your body. I try to remind my trainees that if you don't force your body to change then it will fight like a son of a bitch to maintain balance and equilibrium (we call it homeostasis in biology).

You must pick a weight that makes the proper completion of the set as tough as possible. If you fail to do this, if you fail to provide sufficient stimulation, what possible reason does your body have to adapt and develop?

Of course, the flip side is falling into the trap of going too heavy and selecting a weight that makes it impossible to even get close to the correct completion of a given set.

Notice my emphasis on 'correct completion'. Any fool can load up a barbell and bounce it around to hit the prescribed repetitions, but what about form (crucial for both the right muscular and CNS stimulation, and injury prevention) and tempo? All the programmes in this book have prescribed tempos (which you may have noticed change over the course of a macro-cycle) not just because I like to

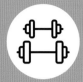

WEIGHT SELECTION SIMPLIFIED

If this is an aspect of training that you feel you struggle with I am going to keep this very simple for you. In this book if you are prescribed an exercise for three sets of 12 reps these are the options available to you:

1 The first set is so easy you could have done 20 reps without breaking sweat. This set doesn't count.

2 The first set you hit a comfortable 12 reps and could have done 15. Wise up – next time when you are at 6 reps and realise it is a bit too easy, stop the set, rest a minute and then resume with a heavier load.

3 The first set you hit a hard 12 reps. Stick with that weight for your next set, but make a note in your training diary and at the next workout you must slightly increase (2–5 per cent) the weight on the opening set of that exercise.

4 You get fewer than 10 reps on your first set – you have started too heavy. Drop the weight by 5–10 per cent for your next set, and consider lightening your starting weight at the next workout, depending on just how heavy that first set felt.

5 As sets progress, if your reps fall to less than 75 per cent of your target reps then drop the weight if there are following sets of that exercise in that workout.

create extra work for myself, but because each of those four numbers changes the stimulus on your muscles for a specific reason. Get it into your head that absolutely everything that you do during a set will affect the quality and magnitude of your results.

Weight selection dictates so much of your response to training that if you get it wrong you may as well kiss goodbye to any sort of tangible progress. If you go too heavy you risk injury, wild form, and an inability to stimulate the right muscle groups. If you go too light then the adaptive response just won't happen because your muscles are not being sufficiently stressed and tested.

HOW TO TRAIN TO GAIN

If 100,000 people buy this book there will probably be 100,000 different interpretations of how to follow the exercise programme. Some of you will attack each repetition, let alone each workout, with a wild abandon (good for you), whereas others will be infinitely more cautious and timid. We will have the guys who lift weights that are far too heavy, and we will have their polar opposites, the ones who always train so far within themselves that they think the programme is rubbish because they haven't changed. No sh*t, Sherlock. If you only do what you can already do, how on earth will your body be stimulated to grow?

One of the key things that distinguishes a successful body transformation is your attitude in the gym. Don't ever hold back. *Intensity of effort – get out of your comfort zone!*

Let's make one thing clear: it is highly unlikely that you can train as hard as me. That's because I have been lifting weights since I was 11 years old, which means I have more than 30 years of training experience. Training intensely is a learned skill. You can't just walk in off the street as a complete beginner and push yourself as hard as a more experienced trainee unless you have a deep and consistent background in physically demanding sports.

However, never use that as an excuse. The only way to learn to train hard is by doing it. That's another reason why you might sense the odd bit of scorn from me for the internet warrior who pontificates but doesn't actually know how to push himself in the gym.

Nor should you despair if you're a beginner and reading these words. Perhaps a better way of expressing what is needed is to say that you need to get out of your comfort zone at each and every workout. You also need to be aware that as you push yourself further along your comfort zone expands. What seemed ball-breakingly tough in your first workout will seem like a walk in the park by your sixth. And this means that you need to constantly keep upping the ante and training harder every time.

STICKING TO THE PLAN

The workout routine in this book has everything in it for a specific reason. As soon as you deviate from the plan the training effect changes. Admittedly some of the workouts may seem complicated if you are used to the fitness fluff of mainstream magazines. Pay close attention to tempo, rest periods and always good exercise form.

FOCUS AND CONCENTRATION

We live in a multimedia age where it is all too easy to be distracted. Even as I write these words I have to resist the pull of social media updates or checking my email. Be smart – don't take your phone into the gym, take an MP3 player instead. Don't chat with your mates, read a magazine, or discuss politics. There's plenty of time to do all that once your hour of training is over.

Successful muscle-building training is all about establishing a strong neurological connection to your muscles, and that only comes with practice and concentration. Furthermore, the best hypertrophy workouts are ones that are done at pace and 'kept alive' with focus and intensity. Keep your eyes on the goal in front of you – it's only four hours a week of training for 12 weeks. There are no excuses.

LIFT WITH INTENT

There are two separate aspects to the meaning of lifting with intent.

First, you don't need to lift a weight up quickly in order for maximum muscle stimulation. You do, however, need to have the intention of lifting up (the concentric component of the contraction) quickly. I want you to try to think this one through because it goes to the heart of much of the overall training experience.

Second, you 'need to lift with intent' like you are moving a dumbbell and not a fairy wand. What I mean here is that before you execute a movement you should know what muscles are supposed to be working and how. When in doubt start lighter and do a few practice sets so that you are better set up to work the right muscles in the right manner when you get to the work sets. When you've got the right set-up and you're locked and loaded, smash out the set with intent on each and every repetition. Don't be dreaming of who's out next in *The X Factor* or colour-coordinating your gym wardrobe with your significant other. In your head, no matter how intimidated you may feel at first in the gym, I want you to train like you own the gym.

DISTINGUISH BETWEEN GOOD AND BAD PAIN

Good training pain is when your muscles shake, your skin feels like it might split because you're so pumped up, and it feels like there's a blowtorch burning the inside of your muscles. This is something that you need to embrace.

Bad pain is sharp joint and/or soft tissue pain that pulls you up short, or a muscle somehow spasming or knotting up so that dysfunction occurs if you carry on. The overwhelming odds are that if you exercise sensibly, always using good form and moving the weight with your muscles and not momentum and leverage, you will never have to experience this.

KEEP A TRAINING DIARY

Any serious trainee who fails to keep a training diary is doing himself a grave disservice and missing out on an array of very easily achieved advantages. If you choose to ignore my advice on this then, if I may be so bold, you are a bit of an idiot. Here's why.

While training progress is never linear we do always want to strive to improve upon what we have done before. If we don't do something more difficult, why would our bodies positively adapt? This becomes especially true as you progress as a trainee because the obvious adaptations, such as increased strength, slow

down, and we need to start manipulating variables such as tempo, rest intervals, joint angles and sets. Unless you are a genius can you really tell me all the reps, sets and weights that you did four weeks ago? I don't think so.

Expanding upon the previous point, a training diary is a motivational tool *par excellence*. Knowing that you have to beat your last session is a massive incentive for most people. Sometimes the physical progress can be hard to properly assess – the mirror hardly ever tells the truth – and using your diary as a way to see how you just keep on getting better will reaffirm everything else that you are doing to change your lifestyle and improve your physique.

DON'T BE A PUSSY

The number one muscle-building commandment in my book is 'Thou shall not be a pussy.'

I don't think I need to add anything more than that but I'll conclude this section with two points that expand on the commandment.

First, ask yourself this question: Will the lion or the lamb dominate in the gym?

Second, when things get tough and you want to quit – something that happens to every single one of us, by the way – remind yourself of the old Schwarzenegger mantra that the gym should be attacked with 'joy and fierceness'. Repeat that in your head when you start to look for a way out. I promise you'll get an extra rep or two out!

04

THE
CARDIO
CONUNDRUM

Cardiovascular exercise is essential for good health, but has a lesser role in achieving better body composition. Indeed, the concept of cardio is completely misunderstood by most.

I f you believe aerobic exercise and cardio are interchangeable terms, or that cardio makes you fat or causes muscle mass to disappear, then you need to read on. The benefits, application and even meaning of 'cardio' require us to go right back to basics because so much confusion has been created by so many so-called experts.

WHAT IT ALL MEANS

The definitions on page 60 illustrate the first problem we have to address in this cardio/aerobic debate – we are pretty much all guilty of using the term cardio training when we really mean aerobic training.

The essence of a 'cardio workout' is that it refers to exercise that is stimulating for our overall cardiovascular system, predominantly the heart. So it stands to reason that anything that maximally exercises the heart and vascular system can count as a cardiovascular training. If you are one of those who associate cardiovascular training as solely belonging to

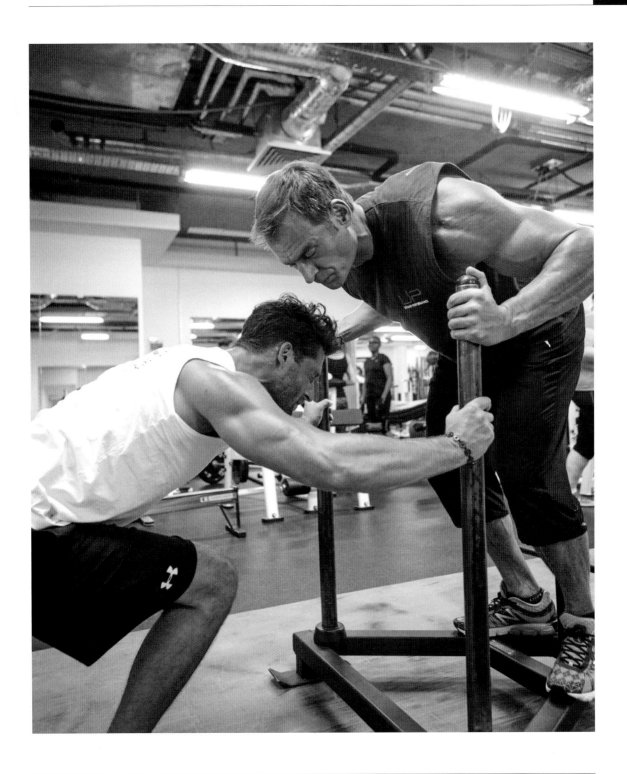

CARDIOVASCULAR EXERCISE

AEROBIC TRAINING

Cardio training is often perceived as being within the exclusive remit of 'aerobic exercise'. Aerobic (meaning 'with oxygen') training is typified by low to moderate levels of exertion, typically over a duration of 20 minutes up to many hours. As a percentage of energy used to fuel the body, fat metabolism is higher than carbohydrate/glycogen metabolism (glycolysis).

However, fewer calories per unit of time are burned than during more intense forms of training (such as anaerobic, meaning 'without oxygen'), and overall metabolic elevation stays higher the more intense the training session.

AEROBIC CAPACITY

Specific aerobic training improves aerobic fitness and aerobic capacity. Aerobic capacity is the functional capacity of the cardiorespiratory system, which is measured by testing VO_2 max, which is an individual's maximum oxygen consumption.

VO_2 max is crucially important for endurance athletes, but of minimal importance to more explosive athletes. Indeed, there is a proven inverse correlation between VO_2 max and an individual's ability to accelerate and explode as measured by a vertical jump. There is also no direct link between VO_2 max and cardiovascular health. This isn't to say that the VO_2 max is useless, or that an improved cardiorespiratory capacity is not a good thing for many people, but it is clearly not the only or even the best way to exercise the heart.

CARDIOVASCULAR HEALTH

The cardiovascular system is one of the most important aspects of our health, and we should pay it constant attention. It is the heart, the veins and the blood vessels, and it takes in pulmonary, systemic and coronary circulation. It has nothing to do with aerobic capacity, which should make you wonder why aerobic training is so commonly conceived as being the only way to exercise for a healthy heart.

CARDIORESPIRATORY FITNESS

Cardiorespiratory fitness is the ability of both the respiratory and the circulatory systems to supply oxygen to skeletal muscles during physical activity. This isn't an asset just for an exercise regime, but also for living a vigorous and fulfilling life. A large number of people seem to believe that cardiorespiratory fitness can only be achieved by aerobic training. Indulge me and let's wonder if there are any other exercise modalities that might vigorously pump blood to skeletal muscles and train the heart ...

the world of the treadmill or stationary bike, stop for a second and ask yourself whether any other forms of exercise might also stimulate the heart.

Some people will tell you that aerobic training is a must for cardiovascular health, regardless of whether an individual weight trains or not. I have even heard medical doctors come out with this line of BS, which is quite staggering. The solution to such ignorance is to teach via experience, and one session into the delights of weight training for fat loss and body composition purposes soon sees them reverse that opinion.

In such circumstances it isn't absolutely necessary to have them gasping for breath, heart beating so hard that our receptionist at the front desk can hear it, vomiting in the sick bucket, and collapsing in a corner of the gym for 50 minutes, but it does give a certain satisfaction as a lesson well learned! What we should all love about resistance training is that it is the most malleable training tool available to us. We can pretty much literally train for any goal that we want.

So if you are gearing up for a power-lifting world record with long slow sessions of triples and a work-to-rest ratio of 10 seconds to seven minutes, then yes, you would certainly benefit from some form of 'cardio training', although this should not be traditional aerobic work but rather some brief modified strongman sessions on the super yoke, farmer's walk and prowler.

On the other hand, the type of training that most people want, the type that adds a sculpted look to the body, very often involves minimal rest periods and a constantly elevated heart rate, all of which are cardio healthy.

WHAT THIS MEANS FOR *YOU*

It means that there are innumerable exercise options open to you if you want to build cardiovascular health. A bit of (hard) aerobic training can be good, and so can some (hard) weight training. Coasting on a stationary bike will have negligible effect, as will weight training the way most people seem to do it in a commercial gym. Sitting yourself down in some fancy machine and lifting a weight for 12 reps that you could actually lift for 100 reps, and then resting five minutes while you text your friends and stare into space, simply does not cut it.

It isn't all that complicated. You just have to work hard! However, if push comes to shove, is there an optimal form of training for cardiovascular health?

The answer to that is a definite affirmative, and it lies squarely in the realm of resistance training. If you are lucky enough to have access to modified strongman training equipment or can train in a gym where super-setting large compound movements is feasible, then you have the ideal cardiovascular training modality.

If you still need convincing, allow me to throw a little bit of science into the mix. There are countless studies proving that left ventricular function of the heart is one of the key predictors of cardiovascular health, and guess what sort of person these studies say have the best ejection fraction and diastolic function? Yes, individuals who regularly practise vigorous resistance training!

Your Honour, I rest my case.

If you want a fantastic bang-for-your-buck routine then try this very simple workout and tell me your heart is not working overtime. This is certainly not your bog-standard cardio training programme, and if you are reasonably well trained and can generate a good degree of force then this will smash you up beyond belief. And your cardiovascular system will benefit from the workout of your life!

Workout A*	Exercise	Sets	Reps	Tempo	Rest	Page
A1	Deadlift	4	10 max	4010	10 secs	89
A2	Standing barbell shoulder press	4	10 max	3010	10 secs	135
A3	Shoulder-width pull-up	4 (add weight if necessary)	10 max	3010	10 secs	136
A4	Back squat	4	10 max	4010	2–4 mins	78

*If you feel this circuit in your lower back then a great alternative is to substitute a regular barbell with a Watson trap bar to shift the emphasis onto the quadriceps.

THE LIES SOME TRAINERS TELL ABOUT 'CARDIO'

Twenty-five years ago, when I was still a teenage boy, I would let a lot of things bother me. Righteous indignation was a common occurrence, and my father used to constantly liken me to a coiled spring. I've mellowed a fair bit since then, but every now and again I allow the red mist to descend and I'll take vehement umbrage at sub-educational idiocy. The politics of imbeciles and training opinions of morons who masquerade as fitness professionals are my two most emotive *bêtes noires.*

A little while ago my slow burn was sparked into fire by a headline I read on social media by some bandwagon-jumping clown. This joker had hitched his colours to the anti-cardio mast and decided to preach that running will make you fatter and that if you exercise near anything electric you are wasting your time.

I am not exaggerating in the slightest.

I am not a huge fan of cardio training, and especially some forms of running, as an optimal body composition tool, but to suggest that if I go for a run I'll get fatter flies in the face of sense and experience.

The fool who writes a headline like 'Run Yourself Fatter' is trying to grab your attention, but what he fails to realise is that most people pick up on just 10 per cent of any message, so no matter what else he may have written most people will only recall the headline.

Mistakes such as these are often compounded by the fallacious argument, one I have heard so often from a certain type of personal trainer, that all you need to do is go to the gym and observe those who weight train and those who do cardio training to see who is the leanest, because it will be the weight trainers who win.

I am willing to bet that I have been in more hardcore weight-training gyms than 99.99 per cent of all personal trainers, and in my experience the fat bastards all tend to congregate around the bench-press platforms and avoid cardio like the plague. And then when they want to lean up, they jump on a treadmill.

This does not mean that these chaps (it's almost always the guys, by the way) are porky because they like to bench press and avoid any form of cardiovascular training; causality is not so simple. But to the eye of the layman, who can observe the lean cardio bunnies and the squidgy weight-lifters, it makes no sense whatsoever and serves to undermine otherwise sensible messages.

Being constructive, let's address where cardio training sits in the pantheon of exercise modalities. It does have a place, and if you do it you won't lose all your muscle! You may have noticed that those who say you will shrink from cardio tend to have very little muscle mass of their own anyway.

Nor will cardio make you fat. Now this shocking revelation is out of the way I am going to list a number of points that you can use to help form your own way of dealing with the cardio conundrum.

14 COMMON SENSE CARDIO TRAINING RULES

01 Cardio is not the best way to get lean if you have limited exercise time. Intensive weight training will always win out if you can only get to the gym three times a week and have zero other opportunities to train.

02 Cardio is a great fat-loss tool for those of you who can only make the gym three to four times a week (for weight training), but have time to exercise at home and/or outdoors on other occasions. My attitude is, why waste good gym time by doing cardio?

03 Long bouts of cardio training can be counterproductive. I don't believe for a second it will make you fatter, but it will negatively impact your cortisol levels, make recovery harder, and be harmful for those of you wanting improved muscle mass or just so-called tone and shape. Basically, extended endurance-style cardio performed repeatedly will make you look 'stringy', and without decent quality muscle you run the risk of becoming the dreaded 'skinny fat'.

04 Aerobic work plateaus after six to eight weeks of training. This means that there is limited value in doing traditional aerobic-style training as a means of continuously improving your fitness. Here is a hint: You can exercise your heart (the true meaning of cardio work as opposed to aerobic training), elevate your metabolism and improve aerobic fitness without an over-emphasis on cardio. In fact, you don't necessarily need any 'traditional cardio' at all. Also, if you do want to do cardio for fat loss and/or fitness, then mixing it up a lot will help prevent your body entering a more efficient, less metabolism-boosting mode. Different machines, different paces, uphill, downhill – the options at your disposal are endless and infinitely better for both mind and body than mindlessly trudging away at the same level.

05 You will hear some people harp on about the oxidative stress and elevated cortisol issues that come with performing cardio. I say if it makes you feel good, and you are otherwise healthy, then a little bit will not hurt you. But this doesn't mean two hours a day, every day, on the treadmill. Hard cardio, be it interval training or steady state, should be done judiciously, but a couple of 30-minute sessions a week will usually only serve to benefit a fat-loss programme, and if you enjoy and feel good when taking a nice long walk then go for it. The positives will far outweigh the negatives. Just don't fool yourself into thinking this is a replacement for the more effective forms of fat-loss training.

06 If you are seeking to maximise muscle mass then 30 minutes of fast walking three times per week may be useful, but is probably not essential if you are weight training hard and with sufficient volume and frequency. A few fast walks on top of four times per week weight training will not really hinder your recovery process unless you have the testosterone levels of a neutered hamster.

07

If you are seeking to maximise muscle mass while getting leaner at the same time then I'd advise a 6:1 ratio of weight training to fast walking. This is a very personal thing, though, and really has a lot to do with your own recovery levels, any calorie deficit, and the type of resistance training protocols you adhere to. If you have limited gym time then you may benefit, for very brief periods when you are focusing on fat loss, in learning a lesson from bodybuilding and adding an extra cardio session three to six times per week separate from your weight training.

08

You must always adapt the training tool to the goal. I do not really like interval training as cardio for those who are primarily concerned with muscle growth or muscle retention. I think the energy demands, both physical and mental, of hard weight training are too great to add interval training on top. If a lean and athletic body is your goal then adding interval training can be a huge benefit, and for most regular people with non-physique competing goals this would be my preferred cardio of choice (after point 14).

09

There is a correct time to perform cardio. If you are going to do all your training in just one session, always perform cardio after your weight training, as the other way around will hinder your lifting performance and limit the fat-burning effectiveness of the cardio: many more fatty acids will be freed up into the bloodstream for energy after weight training than before.

10

Some folk will tell you that you shouldn't perform any cardio training on machines that use electricity as they produce electro-magnetic stress (EMS) that can raise cortisol and induce insulin resistance. And it gets worse, as you shouldn't even be near something as seemingly innocuous as an iPod while training, as it will similarly restrict your fat-loss efforts. I've seen the EMS and hormonal fluctuations study on this and I don't dispute a very mild effect, but let's get a grip. If you are training for the Olympics, then ditch the electrical machines while training. But if not, don't worry about it. The bottom line is that if listening to your iPod inspires you to push harder then by all means go for it.

11 I think the stationary bike is almost as much a waste of time as the recumbent bike! A treadmill, a rowing machine, a versa climber or a punching bag and boxing pads would be my preferred gym tools. All allow for versatile training modalities, and you can cruise or go hard depending upon the circumstances.

12 The best form of steady-state or relatively undemanding cardio training is a brisk walk in the great outdoors. If you haven't tried it for a while I urge you to do so. It will make you feel more alive. It is my personal favourite.

13 If you are a cardio junkie and you are trying to cut down but miss the endorphin rush or runner's high, learn how to weight train using high volume and minimal rest between sets. Find a gym that will be quiet enough to allow a massive giant set circuit – full-body or body-part split, either is good depending upon your goals – and knock yourself out.

14 The absolute best form of fat-burning, fitness-enhancing cardio training isn't really what most people consider to be cardio at all. If I were to supplement any type of fat loss and/or conditioning regime with extra training sessions above and beyond a tough resistance training regime it would be by adding in modified strongman training. The beautiful thing about this training modality is that it elevates the metabolism and keeps it elevated for up to 36 hours; it allows you to train in a truly functional and primal manner that traditional cardio on machines can never do; there is minimal impact and repetition in comparison to running; it is so much easier on soft tissue; and it is so challenging and so much fun!

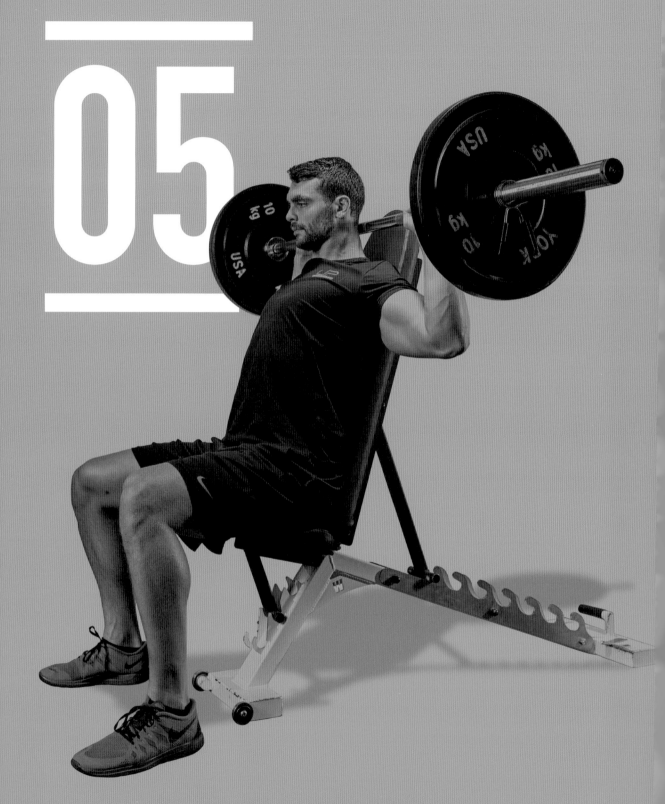

05

THE ULTIMATE BODY TRANSFORMATION WORKOUT PLAN

You've graduated from the entry-level workouts (on pages 33 and 62) and are now ready to tackle the core programme of this book.

Y ou probably want the 12-week programme laid out for you step by step, day by day. My apologies, but this plan doesn't quite work like that. To help you create a routine that suits your own very specific goals I have constructed a workout regime that allows you to add and subtract routines based on the areas of your body that you want to give special attention to. For example, if you have arms like wet linguini then you need to do additional arms work. If you're a narrow beanpole then you need to do extra shoulder work.

The more effort, more volume and more intensity we apply to a muscle the more it will respond, up to a point.

THE WORKOUTS

The ideal scenario is that we temporarily overload the muscle, often called *overreaching*, and then we back off to allow supercompensation (a positive rebound) to occur.

However, we must always bear in mind that the human body can only tolerate so

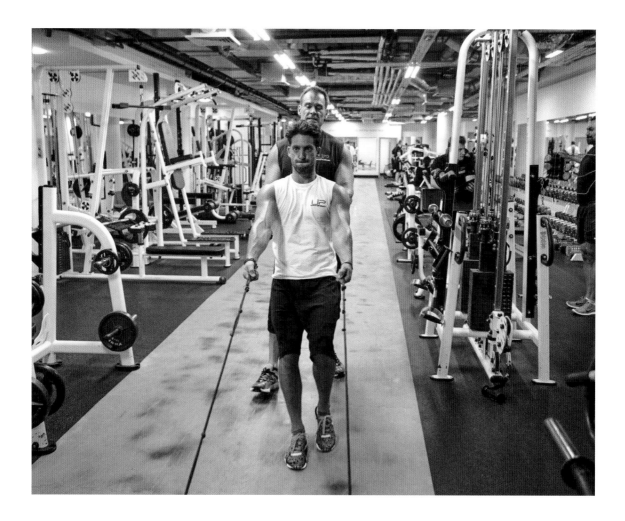

much work and stress before the training becomes counterproductive. This is commonly referred to as *overtraining*. If you reach the overtraining stage then the only recourse is rest and recuperation until you get back to normal. You've gone too far and are unlikely to experience the benefits of supercompensation.

The routines that you will follow factor all this in to give you the following:

- A foundation 12-week programme that you consistently follow.
- Specialisation routines that allow you to give extra attention to specific body parts.
- Enforced back-off periods to allow supercompensation and maximum muscle growth.

THE WORKOUT ESSENTIALS FOR YOUR OWN PERSONAL PLAN

it is more than enough for those areas of your body that you are happy to see slower improvements with while focusing more effort, and frequency, on lagging body parts.

Therefore, every week you will **follow two of the three Foundation Workouts only. Let me make that clear – you do not do all three weekly Foundation Workouts.**

Why? Because you will drop one of the three sessions and replace it with two sessions from the Specialisation Workouts.

SPECIALISATION WORKOUTS

You have the option of specialising on your arms, chest, shoulders, back and legs.

If you want to pay extra attention to your abs then there's a 99.9 per cent chance that you need to prioritise getting leaner and not building them up, which is why I have left them out of the book to avoid an unnecessary distraction. If you do fall into that 0.1 per cent then the specialisation routines are available as a free download at www.UltimateTransformation.Guide.

Each specialisation routine is numbered A to E or A to F (depending on the split) and lasts for three weeks. It must be followed for the duration, and only ever do one specialisation routine at a time.

You can specialise on the same muscle group more than once in the 12-week programme, but you must not do them consecutively. You must always have a three-week gap in between where you specialise on another body part.

FOUNDATION WORKOUTS

The Foundation Workout plan contains three sessions per week for each of the 12 weeks. Numbered 1 to 36, these three weekly sessions each focus on different muscle groups: one is chest and back; one is legs; and the final one is arms and delts.

If you followed only this plan you would get some great workouts in but you would only be training your main muscle groups once per week. This frequency of stimulus is too low for maximum results. However,

For example, if chest and arms are your only priorities you could follow the workout specialisation strategy below. You will find detailed step-by-step guides to all the exercises in the Foundation and Specialisation Workouts in the next section.

HOW TO MAINTAIN

The beauty of the 12-week training plan in this book isn't just that you can specialise and prioritise different muscles to build a better, bigger and more balanced body; it's that the programme can essentially be followed for the rest of your training days. That's because once you have completed the 12-week programme you can simply return to the beginning and start again. You'll need to increase the weights you lift to keep your muscles growing – which won't be a problem, because you will be significantly stronger – then you can simply add in the Specialisation Workouts for those muscle groups you now need to focus on and improve. Say you focused on delts and arms for the first 12 weeks, like we did with Joe; start again and now focus on your chest and back, or your legs, or whatever muscle group you want to build. And you can repeat this strategy again and again to keep getting bigger, stronger and leaner. That's why this book is the only training guide you'll ever need.

WEEKS 1–3

Arms Specialisation
+
Foundation Weeks 1–3
Chest and Back, Legs
(Arms and Delts would be dropped from the Foundation Workouts)

WEEKS 4–6

Chest Specialisation
+
Foundation Weeks 4–6
Arms and Delts, Legs
(Chest and Back would be dropped from the Foundation Workouts)

WEEKS 7–9

Arms Specialisation
+
Foundation Weeks 7–9
Chest and Back, Legs
(Arms and Delts would be dropped from the Foundation Workouts)

WEEKS 10–12

Chest Specialisation
+
Foundation Weeks 10–12
Arms and Delts, Legs
(Chest and Back would be dropped from the Foundation Workouts)

STEP-BY-STEP EXERCISE FORM GUIDE

Before we get into the detail of the workouts, I'm going to take you through all the exercises step by step, giving you handy tips on how to get the most out of each exercise. Remember, it's about placing maximum stress on your muscle fibres in order to stimulate the most powerful muscle growth. All of the exercises in this section are included in the Foundation and Specialisation Workouts.

SEE IT, SHAZAM IT!

For more detail on all of the exercises in this section you can use the Shazam app on your smart phone. In each exercise, look for the image with the and Shazam it to instantly unlock an exclusive video demonstration with commentary.

Download the Android and Apple app from Shazam.com or the App store.

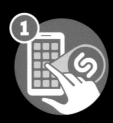

OPEN
the Shazam app

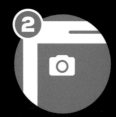

TAP
the camera
icon in Shazam

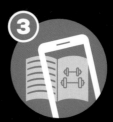

POINT
at anything
with to unlock
more

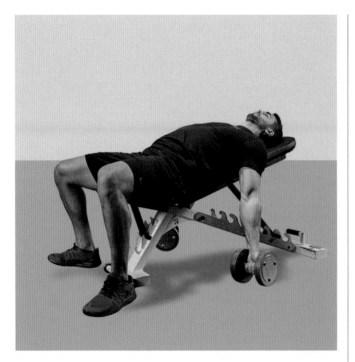

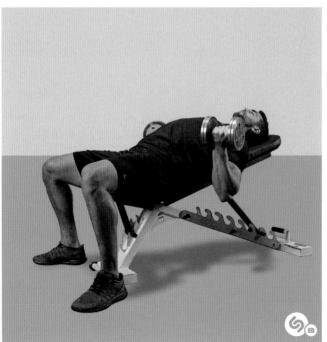

30° DUMBBELL CURL

01 Sit on a 30° incline bench holding a dumbbell in each hand.

02 Keeping your back flat against the bench and your elbows close to your sides, curl the weights up to shoulder height.

03 Squeeze your biceps at the top of the move.

04 Slowly return to the start.

✚

NICK'S TIP

Contract your triceps as hard as possible at the bottom of the movement (under control, do not bounce it!), and squeeze at the top as if you're trying to squash a pencil in the crook of your arm.

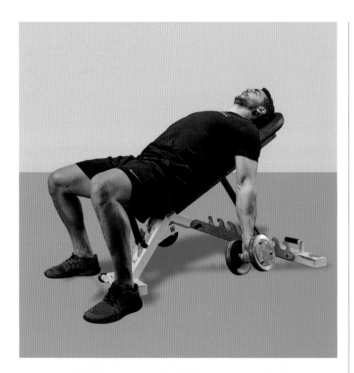

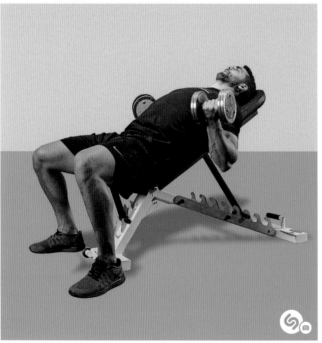

45° DUMBBELL CURL

01 Sit on a 45° incline bench holding a dumbbell in each hand.

02 Keeping your back flat against the bench and your elbows close to your sides, curl the weights up to shoulder height.

03 Squeeze your biceps at the top of the move.

04 Slowly return to the start.

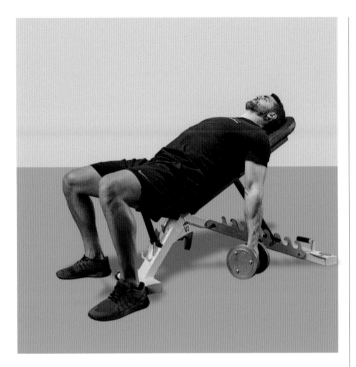

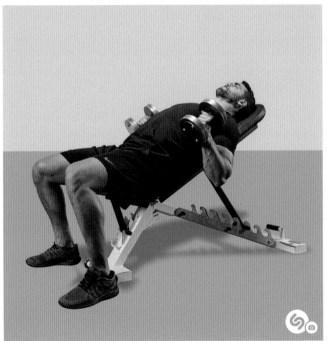

60° HAMMER CURL

01 Sit on a 60° incline bench holding a dumbbell in each hand with palms facing.

02 Keeping your back flat against the bench and your elbows close to your sides, curl the weights up to shoulder height.

03 Squeeze your biceps at the top of the move.

04 Slowly return to the start.

+

NICK'S TIP

Resist the urge to rest the dumbbells on the top of your shoulders in the fully contracted position.

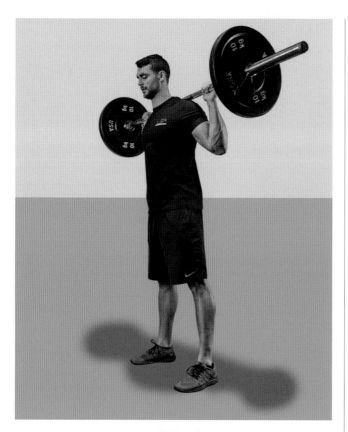

BACK SQUAT

01 Stand tall with your chest up, with a barbell resting on the top of your shoulders, held with an overhand grip.

02 Keeping your chest up and core braced, squat down until your thighs are at least parallel to the floor.

03 Powerfully return to the start.

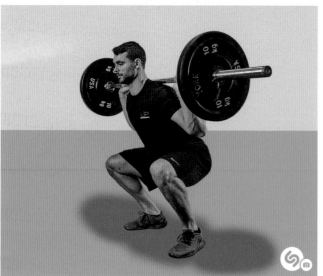

+

NICK'S TIP

Elevating the heels with a board will help 95 per cent of trainees adopt better squatting form. A second tip is to brace hard and squeeze the bar down over your shoulders throughout the movement.

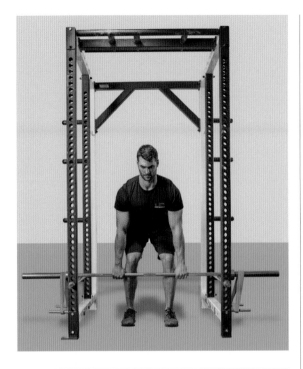

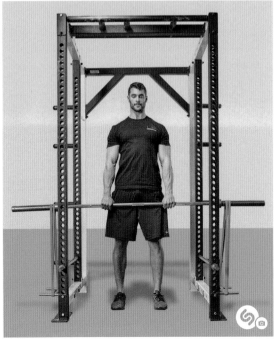

BAND DEADLIFT

01   Stand in a squat rack in front of a barbell with a band attached on each side of the bar to a pin.

02   Squat down to grip it with an overhand grip just outside your knees.

03   Keeping your core braced and your shoulders retracted, push down through your heels to lift the bar up.

04   Keep the bar close to your body and, as it passes your knees, push your hips forward.

05   Reverse the movement back to the start.

✛ NICK'S TIP

In your training programme we're doing this exercise for increased mid and upper back activation. This means that you should take a wide grip, at least 6 inches wider than each shoulder, and focus on keeping your shoulderblades pulled back as hard as possible throughout the entire lifting phase. You will also benefit from using some lifting straps on this exercise so that your grip doesn't become the weak link.

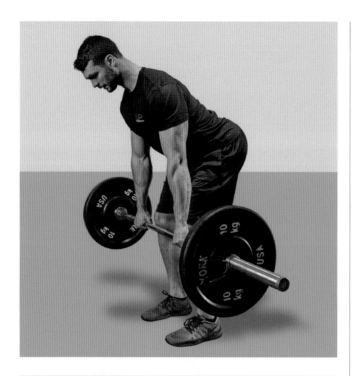

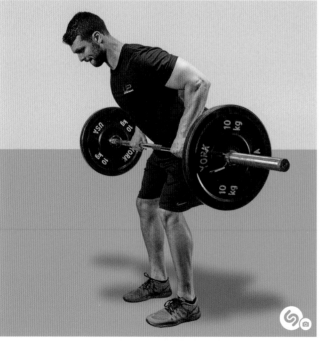

BARBELL BENT-OVER ROW

01 Stand tall with your chest up holding a barbell with an overhand grip slightly wider than shoulder-width apart.

02 Bend your knees slightly and lean forward from the hips, keeping your core braced.

03 Pull the bar up into your belly button, leading with your elbows.

04 Slowly lower the bar to return to the start.

✚

NICK'S TIP

With this exercise it's all too easy for good form to go out of the window in the quest to lift heavier weights. Focus on the contraction and keeping the elbows tight into the body through the lift. If you can't do that then lighten the weight.

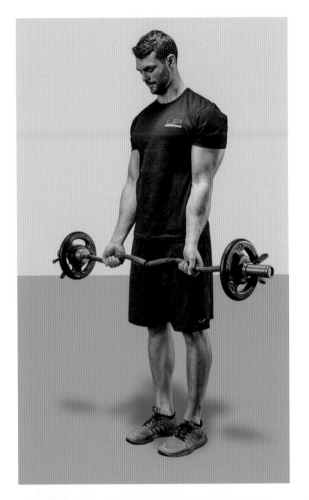
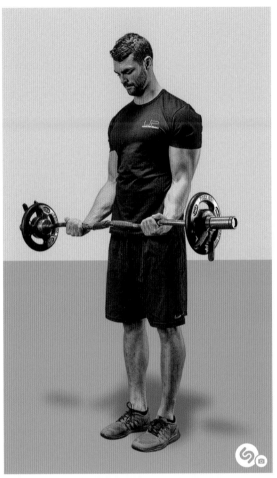

BARBELL WRIST CURL

01 Stand with your chest up holding a barbell with an underhand grip.

02 Curl your wrists up towards your forearm.

03 Slowly return to the start.

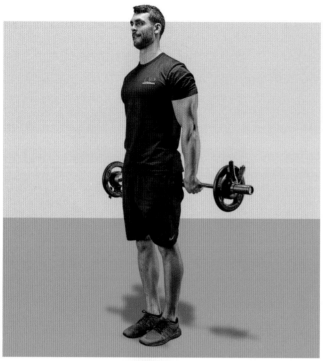

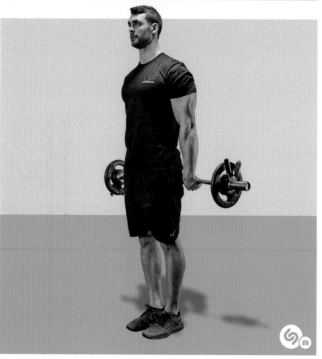

BEHIND BACK BARBELL WRIST CURL

01 Stand with your chest up holding a barbell behind your back with palms facing behind you.

02 Curl your wrists up towards your forearms.

03 Slowly return to the start.

NICK'S TIP

Small movements like this are easy to rush, so be wary. Instead milk every rep by ensuring that you curl your wrists up as far as they will go at the peak contraction point.

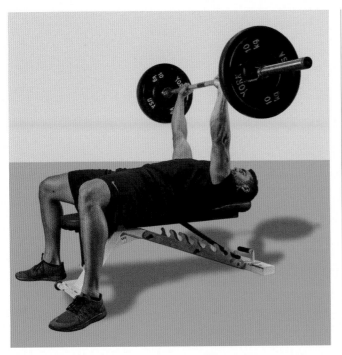

BENCH PRESS

01 Lie on a flat bench with your feet on the floor, directly underneath your knees.

02 Hold the bar with an overhand wide grip.

03 Slowly lower the bar to your chest, until it almost touches your nipples.

04 Press back strongly to the start.

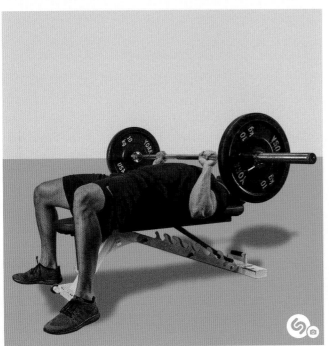

+

NICK'S TIP

Do not bounce the weight off your chest; squeeze your shoulderblades back and down on the negative (lowering) part of the rep; tuck your elbows in so that your upper arms are at about 60 degrees to the torso.

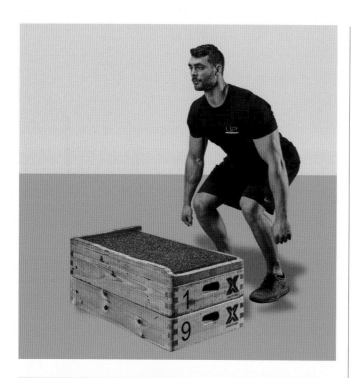

BOX JUMP

01 Stand in front of a box.

02 Bend down and jump explosively up onto the box.

03 Step back down to the start position.

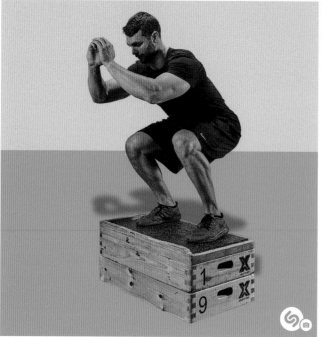

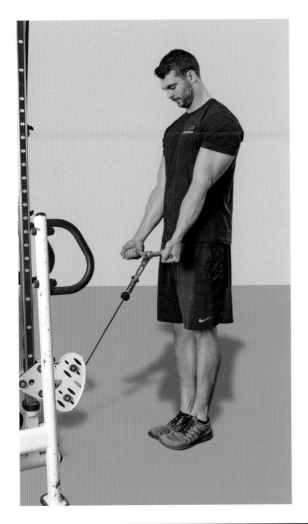
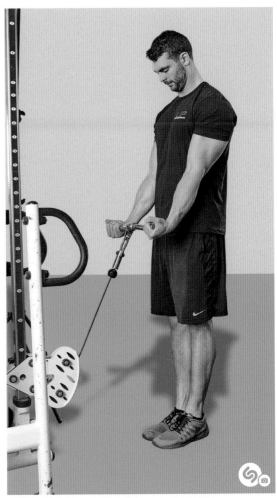

CABLE WRIST CURL

01 Stand tall facing a cable machine with a bar behind your back, attached to the low pulley, with your palms facing away.

02 Curl your wrists up towards your forearm.

03 Slowly return to the start.

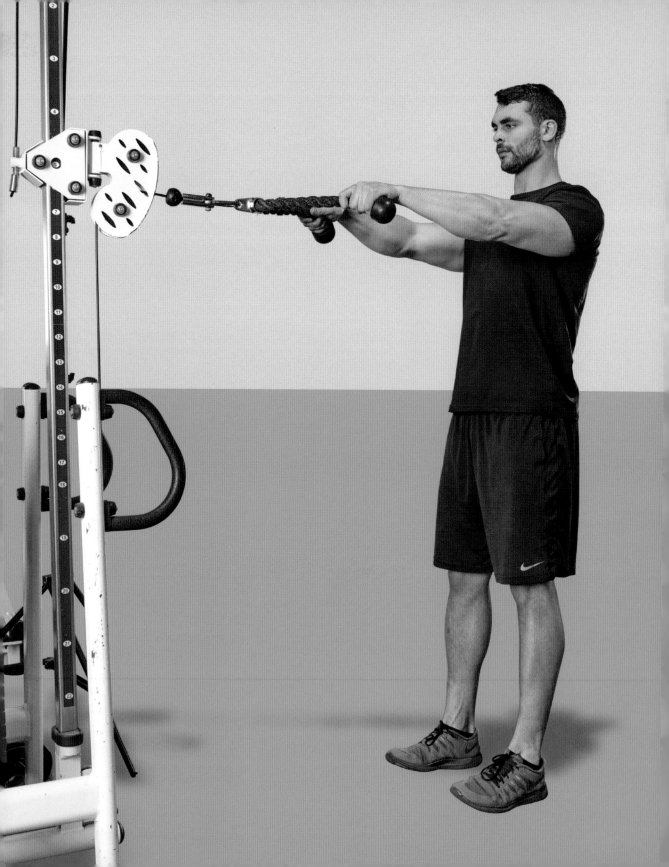

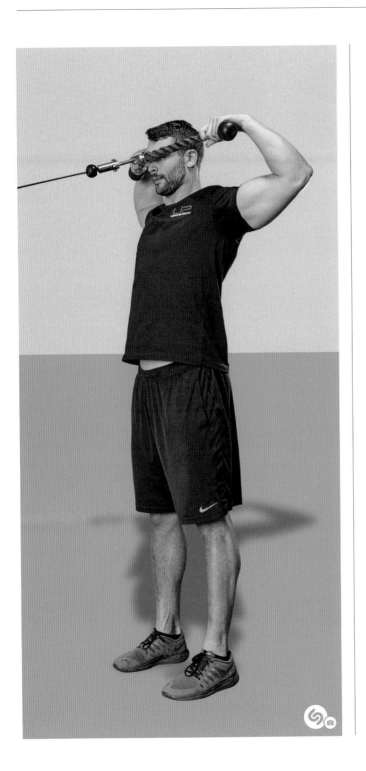

CABLE FACE PULL

01   Attach and hold a double-rope attachment to the high pulley on a cable machine.

02   Pull the handles towards your head, keeping your upper arms parallel to the floor, so that each handle goes either side of your face.

03   Slowly return to the start.

+

NICK'S TIP

If you struggle to feel this movement standing up, even when using a split stance, then try leaning against something solid or even sitting down. This will better help you to isolate the upper back and posterior deltoids.

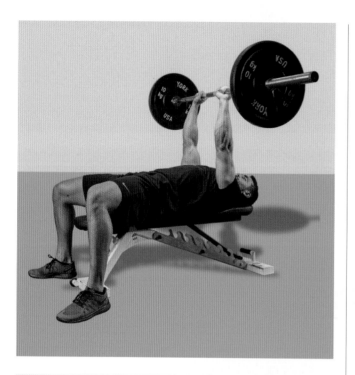

CLOSE-GRIP BENCH PRESS

01 Lie on a flat bench with your feet on the floor, directly underneath your knees.

02 Hold the bar with an overhand shoulder-width grip.

03 Slowly lower the bar to your chest, until it almost touches your nipples.

04 Press back strongly to the start.

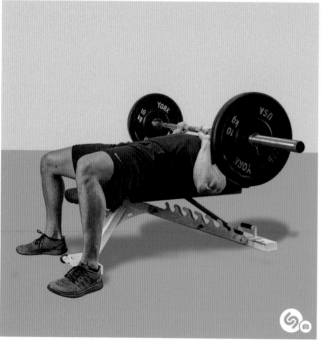

+

NICK'S TIP

Don't take such a close grip that your wrists take the strain. Typically the best grip would be with your hands about 12 inches apart.

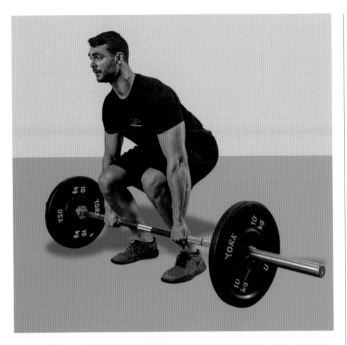

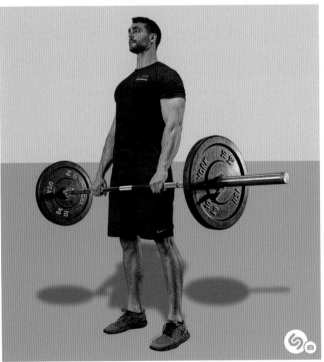

DEADLIFT

01   Stand in front of a barbell and squat down to grip it with either an overhand or alternate grip just outside your knees.

02   Keeping your core braced and your shoulders retracted, push down through your heels to lift the bar up.

03   Keep the bar close to your body and, as it passes your knees, push your hips forward.

04   Reverse the movement back to the start.

✚ NICK'S TIP

Don't lean forward too much by pushing the weight onto the toes; instead sit back a little and then push through the floor. Deadlifting in running trainers is often a bad idea, and stocking feet, if your gym permits it, is often a useful way to improve form.

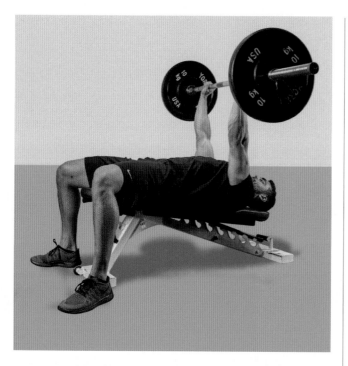

DECLINE BENCH PRESS

01   Lie on a decline bench.

02   Hold the bar with an overhand wide grip.

03   Slowly lower the bar to your chest, until it almost touches your nipples.

04   Press back strongly to the start.

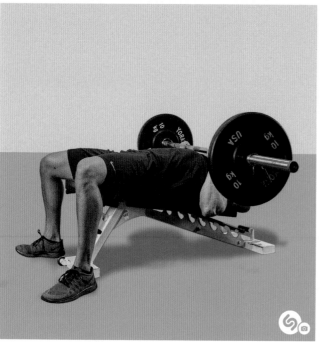

+ NICK'S TIP

You can go heavier on a decline movement than a flat or incline so don't be afraid to load up here as long as form is kept perfect.

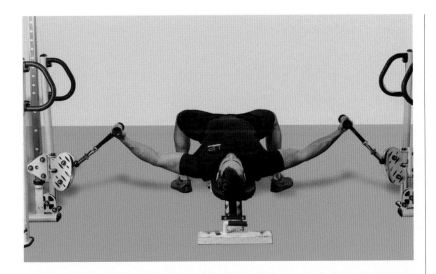

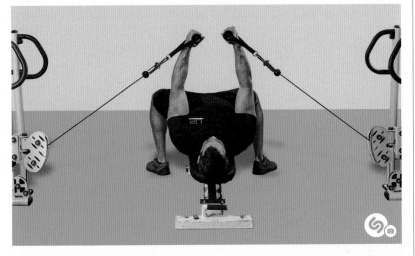

DECLINE CABLE FLYE

01 Lie on a decline bench in the middle of the cable machine, holding a D-handle attached to the low pulley in each hand.

02 Keeping a slight bend in your elbows, raise the handles up and over your chest.

03 Slowly return to the start.

+

NICK'S TIP

For a better contraction internally rotate the elbows so that your thumbs are facing one another. As you fatigue you can then externally rotate to the standard palms facing inward position.

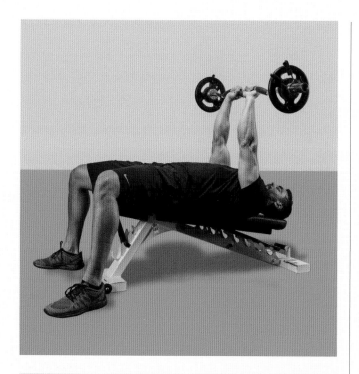

DECLINE CLOSE-GRIP EZ-BAR TRICEPS EXTENSION

01 Lie on a decline bench holding an EZ-bar above your chest with a narrow overhand grip.

02 Slowly lower the bar down towards the top of your head by bending your elbows, but keep them pointing straight up.

03 Slowly return to the start.

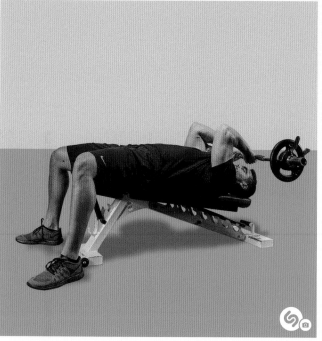

⊕ NICK'S TIP

As long as there is no elbow pain try to keep your elbows tucked in, as opposed to flaring out at the sides, at least until fatigue sets in.

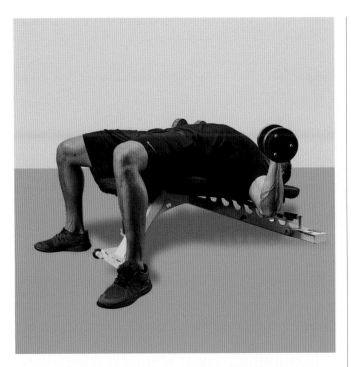

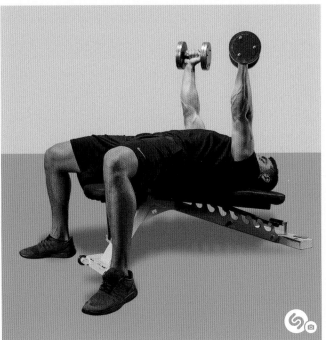

DECLINE DUMBBELL BENCH PRESS

01 Lie on a bench set at a decline angle holding a dumbbell in each hand at shoulder height.

02 Keep your feet flat on the floor and back against the bench.

03 Press the weight straight up.

04 Slowly return to the start.

NICK'S TIP

For the best contraction of your chest muscles think about drawing the upper arms partially across the ribcage at the top of the movement.

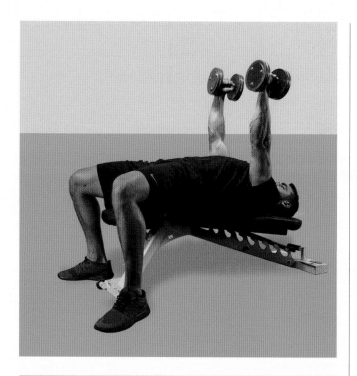

DECLINE DUMBBELL FLYE

01 Lie on a bench set at a decline angle holding a dumbbell in each hand with arms straight.

02 Keep your feet flat on the floor and back against the bench.

03 Keeping a slight bend in your elbow, slowly lower the weights out to the side.

04 Slowly return to the start.

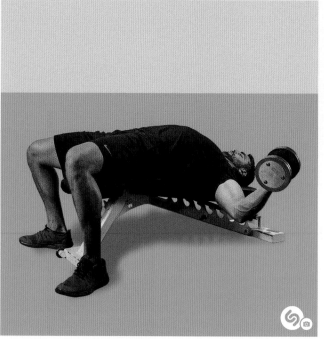

+

NICK'S TIP

Follow Arnold Schwarzenegger's advice on flyes and imagine that you are hugging a giant tree or a beautiful, but very large, woman!

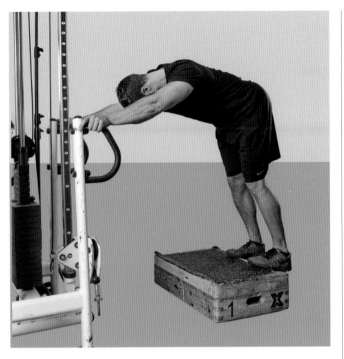

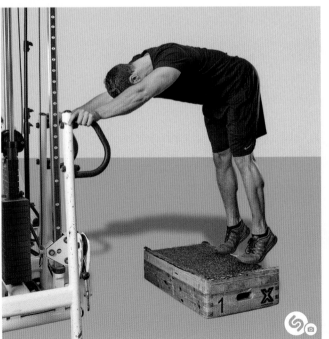

DONKEY CALF RAISE

01 Stand with your toes on a box, bent forward at the hips.

02 Go up on to your tiptoes.

03 Slowly return to the start.

+

NICK'S TIP

If you're strong enough you can have a partner jump on your back, but do take care! Don't underestimate yourself here – think about how much weight one leg takes when running and jumping.

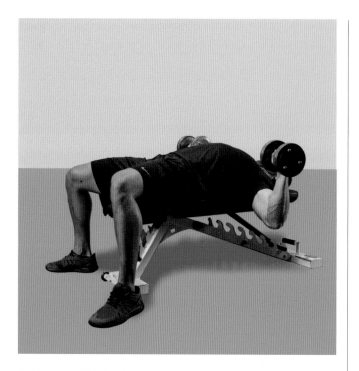

DUMBBELL BENCH PRESS

01 Lie on a flat bench holding a dumbbell in each hand at shoulder height.

02 Keep your feet flat on the floor and upper back against the bench.

03 Press the weight straight up.

04 Slowly return to the start.

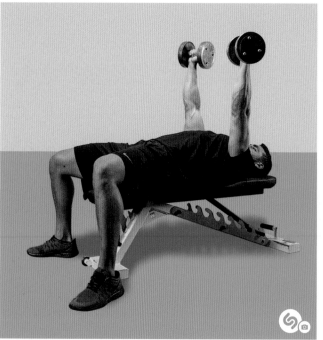

(+)

NICK'S TIP

Squeeze your shoulder-blades back and down as you lower the weight, and as you raise the weight focus on keeping a high ribcage by not pushing through the shoulders.

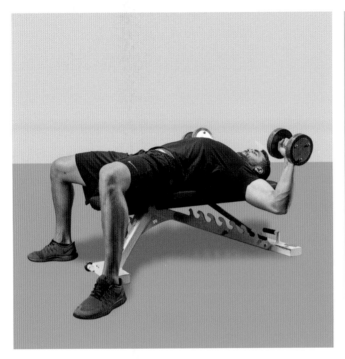

DUMBBELL NECK PRESS

01 Lie on a flat bench holding a dumbbell in each hand either side of your neck.

02 Keep your feet flat on the floor and upper back against the bench.

03 Press the weight straight up.

04 Slowly return to the start.

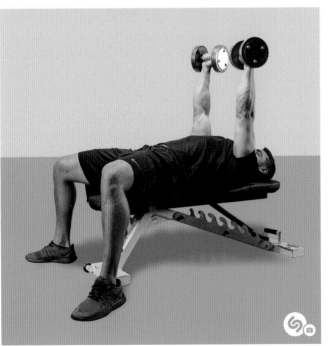

+

NICK'S TIP

You're putting your shoulders in a vulnerable position with this exercise so please don't try to go too hardcore with the weight that you're lifting. Be methodical and controlled, focus on a non-ballistic stretch at the bottom and a hard contraction at the top of each movement.

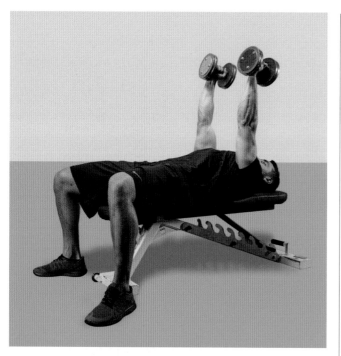

DUMBBELL SKULL-CRUSHER

01 Lie on a flat bench holding a dumbbell in each hand with arms straight.

02 Slowly lower the weights down towards your face by bending your elbows, but keep them pointing straight up.

03 Slowly return to the start.

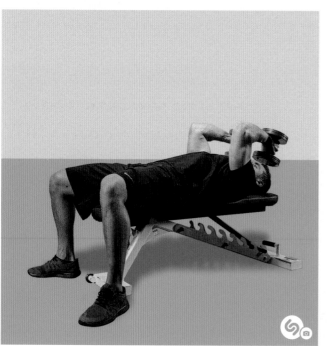

⊕

NICK'S TIP

Only move the weight from the elbow, don't throw it up like you're chucking a ball as far as it will go.

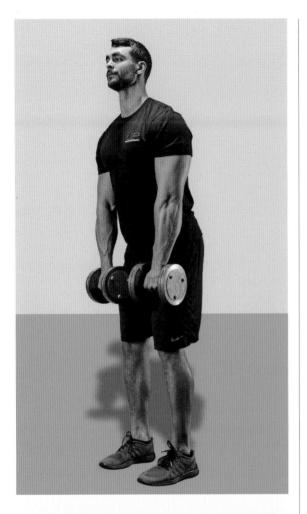

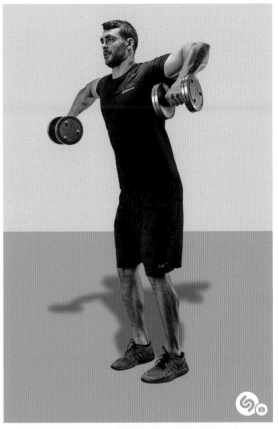

DUMBBELL UPRIGHT ROW

01 Stand with your chest up holding a dumbbell in each hand with an overhand grip.

02 Leading with your elbows, pull the weights up until your hands are level with the top of your chest.

03 Slowly return to the start.

NICK'S TIP

Pull the dumbbells out to your side rather than simply 'up' and in front of your body. It may force you to use a lighter weight but you will hit the all-important side deltoids much more effectively.

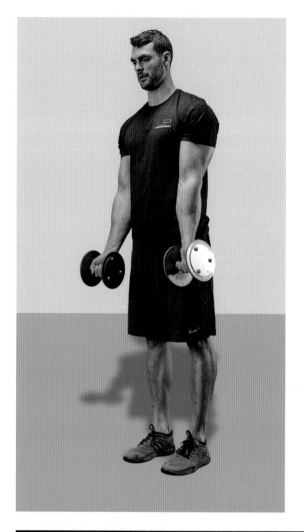
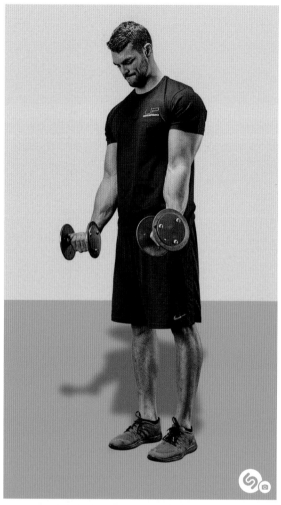

DUMBBELL WRIST CURL

01 Stand with your chest up holding a dumbbell in each hand with palms facing forward.

02 Curl your wrists up towards your forearms.

03 Slowly return to the start.

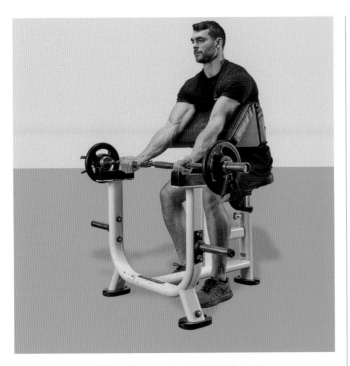

EZ-BAR
PREACHER CURL

01 Sit at a preacher bench holding an EZ-bar with an underhand grip.

02 Keeping your elbows on the bench, curl the bar up towards your chin.

03 Slowly return to the start.

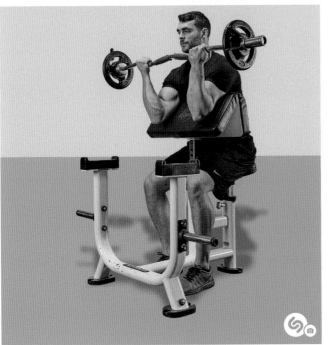

+

NICK'S TIP

Keep your shoulders down throughout the movement rather than lifting them up to the sky. This will better isolate the target biceps muscles.

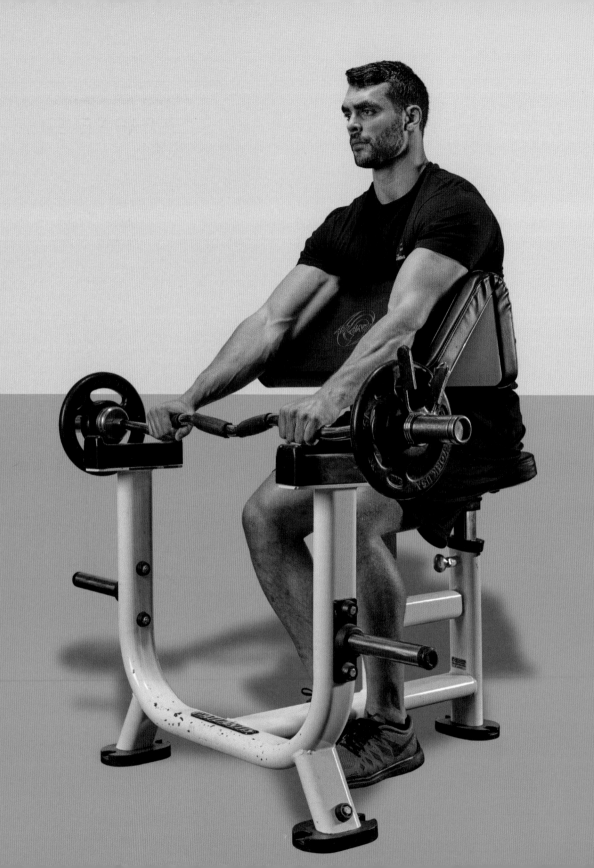

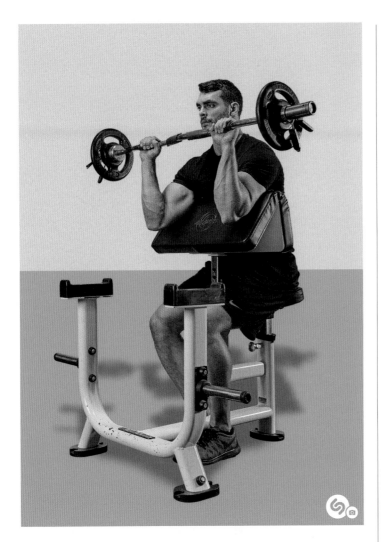

EZ-BAR REVERSE CURL

01   Sit tall with your chest up holding an EZ-bar with an overhand grip.

02   Keeping your elbows by your sides, curl the bar up towards your chin.

03   Slowly return to the start.

+

NICK'S TIP

If you go too heavy your elbows will flare out and the exercise will lose effectiveness. Keep your upper arm locked in tight to your side, and only bend at the elbow rather than also moving from the shoulder to bring the bar up towards the face as this will do nothing other than fatigue your rotator cuff and anterior deltoids.

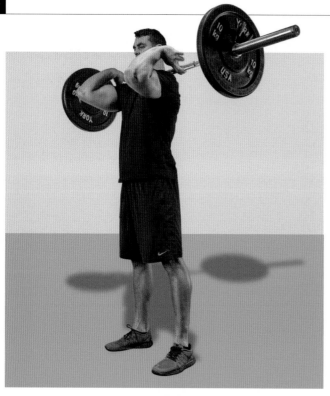

FRONT SQUAT

01 Stand tall with your chest up, with a barbell resting on the front of your shoulders, gripping it with either your elbows pointing forward or your hands crossed in front of your shoulders.

02 Keeping your chest up and core braced, squat down until your thighs are at least parallel to the floor.

03 Powerfully return to the start.

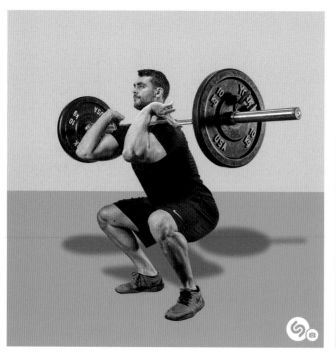

➕

NICK'S TIP

There is no excuse for a full range of motion on this exercise. Ensure that your hamstrings always touch your calves, and if you find yourself going up on your toes as you go down into the squat then elevate the heels on a small board or a pair of 5kg weight plates.

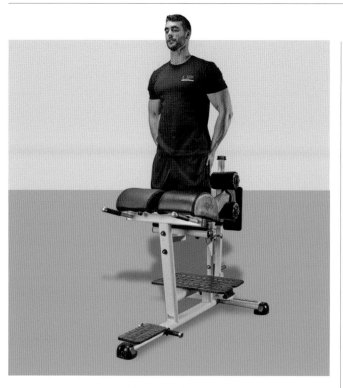

GLUTE-HAM RAISE

01 Following its instructions, position yourself correctly and safely on the machine.

02 Slowly lower your torso down, bending at the hips, until you feel a good stretch in your hamstrings.

03 Powerfully return to the start.

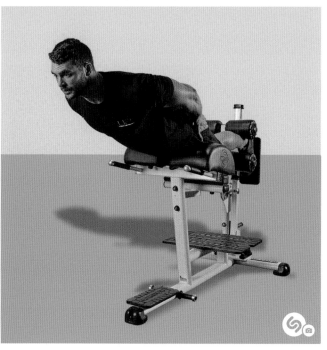

+

NICK'S TIP

If you don't have this machine in your gym then a way to mimic the movement is to do a Nordic curl where a partner holds the back of your legs and from a kneeling position you lower your torso to the floor while locking your hips forwards in extension (i.e. you don't push your buttocks back).

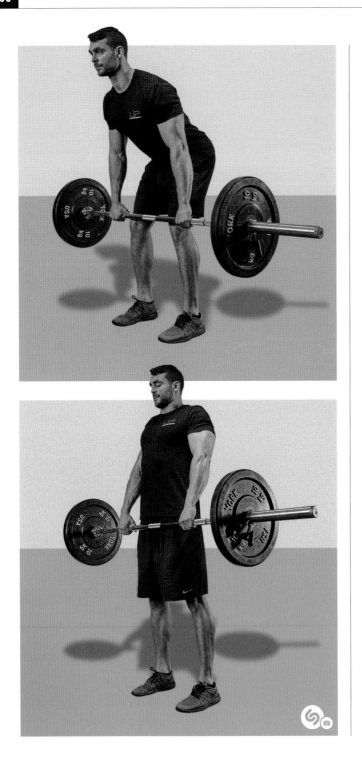

HALF-DEADLIFT WITH SHRUG

01   With the barbell resting on the floor, squat down and take an overhand grip with your core braced, and shoulder-blades retracted.

02   Keeping your core braced, push down through your heels to lift the bar up.

03   Then, keeping your arms straight, shrug the bar up so your shoulders move towards your ears.

04   Reverse back to the start.

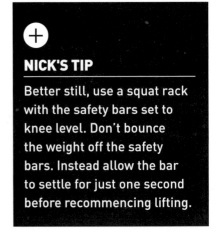

NICK'S TIP

Better still, use a squat rack with the safety bars set to knee level. Don't bounce the weight off the safety bars. Instead allow the bar to settle for just one second before recommencing lifting.

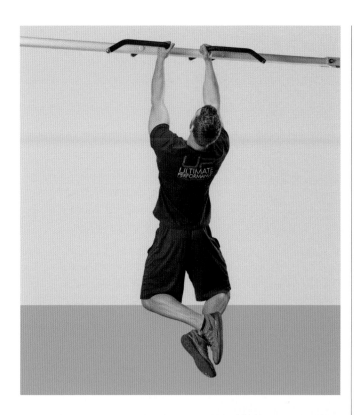

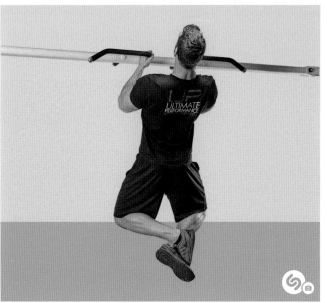

HAMMER-GRIP CHIN-UP

01 Hold the bar with your hands shoulder-width apart and palms facing.

02 Start from a dead hang with your arms fully extended.

03 Pull yourself up so your chin goes over the bar by squeezing your lats.

04 Slowly return to the start.

+

NICK'S TIP

Otherwise known as a semi-supinated grip chin-up, it is easy to bang out a lot of half reps on this movement and very hard to get perfect ones. If you can't get that chest to the bar then there are rotator cuff muscle extras for free download at www. UltimateTransformation. Guide.

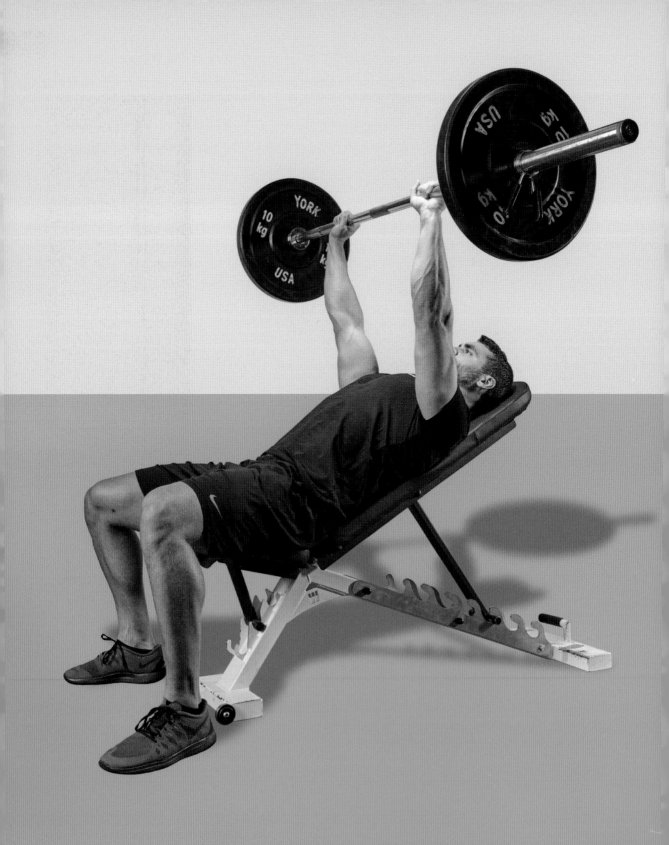

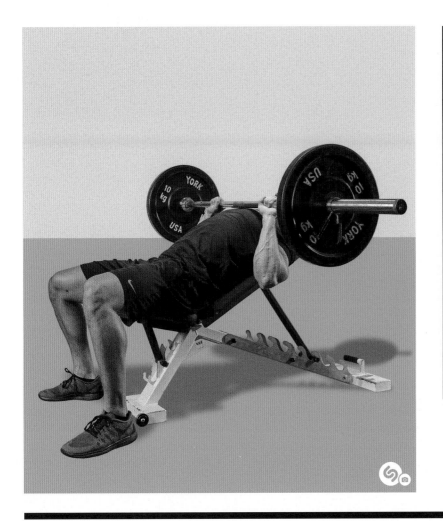

+

NICK'S TIP

Keep your shoulder-blades pushed back and down throughout the whole movement. It is very easy to try to 'force' this movement by pushing through the upper back, and this puts your shoulders in a more vulnerable position.

INCLINE BENCH PRESS

01 Lie on an incline bench with your feet on the floor, directly underneath your knees.

02 Hold the bar with an overhand wide grip.

03 Slowly lower the bar to your chest, until it almost touches your nipples.

04 Press back strongly to the start.

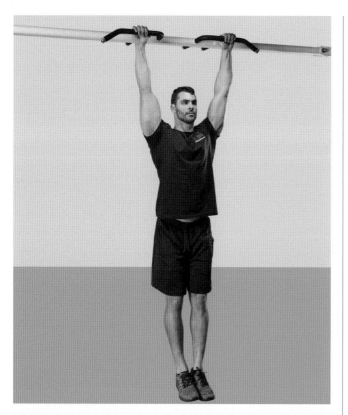

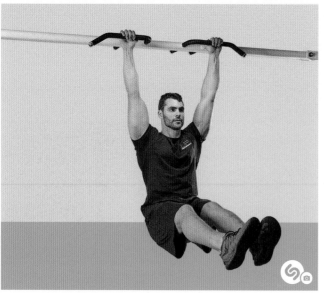

HANGING LEG RAISE

01 Hang from a bar with an overhand grip and your body straight.

02 Keeping your knees locked, use your lower abs to raise your legs up until they are parallel with the ground.

03 Slowly return to the start.

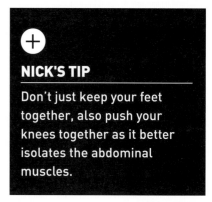

NICK'S TIP

Don't just keep your feet together, also push your knees together as it better isolates the abdominal muscles.

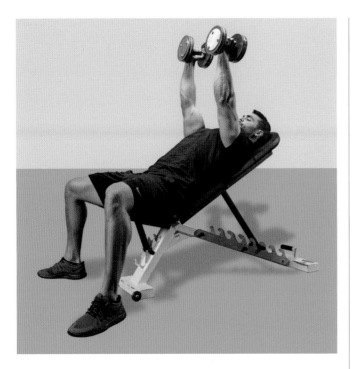

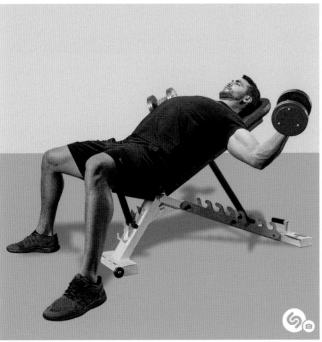

INCLINE DUMBBELL FLYE

01 Lie on a bench set at an incline angle holding a dumbbell in each hand with arms straight.

02 Keep your feet flat on the floor and your back against the bench.

03 Keeping a slight bend in your elbow, slowly lower the weights out to the side.

04 Slowly return to the start.

➕
NICK'S TIP

Your mantra on this movement is to stretch and squeeze. And do it as hard as you possibly can.

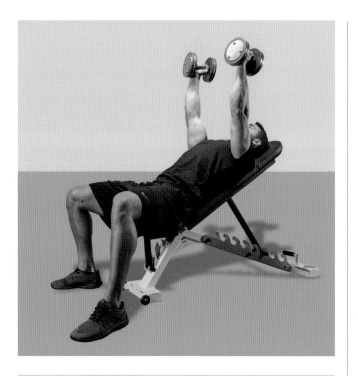

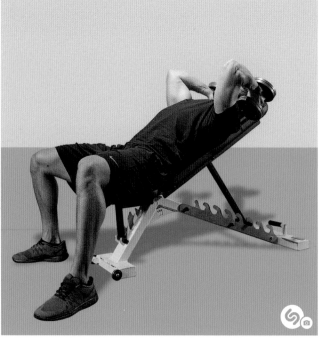

INCLINE DUMBBELL TRICEPS EXTENSION

01 Lie on an incline bench holding a dumbbell in each hand with arms straight.

02 Slowly lower the weights down towards the top of your head by bending your elbows, but keep them pointing straight up.

03 Slowly return to the start.

+ NICK'S TIP

Don't let the elbows flare out too much and do not 'throw' the weight up. Lock the upper arm in one stable position and hold it there, only moving the weight from the elbow joint and not the shoulder.

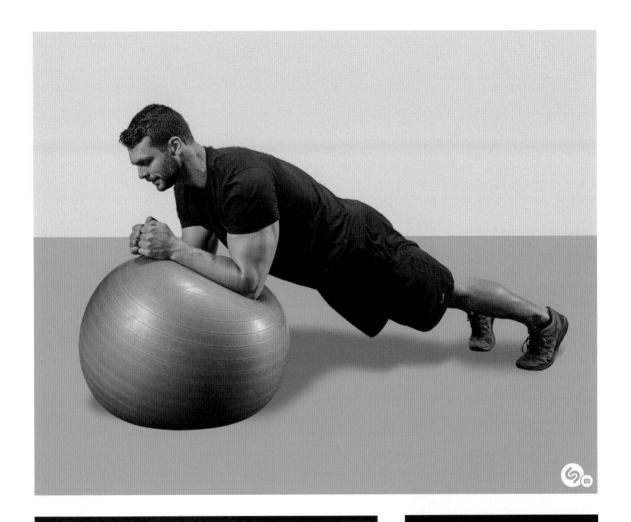

INCLINE GYM BALL PLANK

01 Assume a plank position with your forearms resting on a gym ball with legs straight.

02 Maintain a straight line from head to heels, keeping your core braced and not letting your hips sag.

NICK'S TIP

Squeeze your glutes as hard as possible throughout the entire set. Put a stopwatch on the floor right in front of your eyes so that you can count down (and beat!) your target.

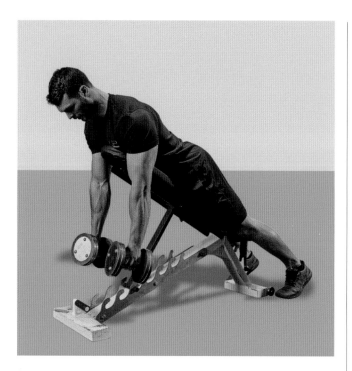

INCLINE REVERSE DUMBBELL ROW

01   Lie chest-first on an incline bench holding a dumbbell in each hand with palms facing.

02   Keeping your chest on the bench, lift the weights up by retracting your shoulderblades, leading with your elbows.

03   Slowly return to the start.

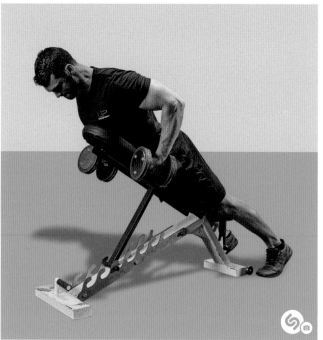

+

NICK'S TIP

You are not merely pulling the weight back with your arms, you are in fact trying to arc your arm back as if you are starting an outboard motor on a boat or a petrol-powered lawn-mower.

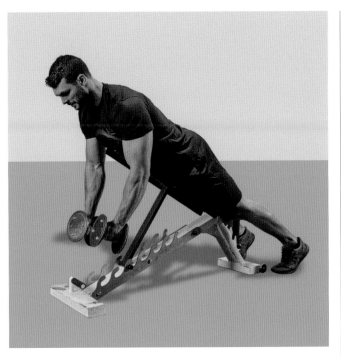

INCLINE REVERSE LATERAL RAISE

01 Lie chest-first on an incline bench holding a dumbbell in each hand with palms facing.

02 Keeping your chest on the bench, lift the weights up and out to the side, keeping a slight bend in your elbows.

03 Slowly return to the start.

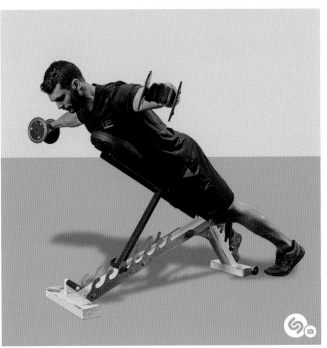

+

NICK'S TIP

Try internally rotating (turning the hands down so that the thumbs point at the floor) the dumbbells to better isolate your rear deltoids.

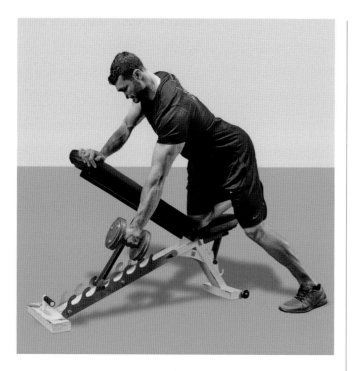

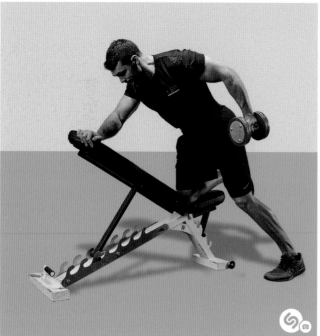

INCLINE REVERSE ONE-ARM ARC ROW

01 Placing your knee and non-working hand on an incline bench for support, hold a dumbbell in one hand with the palm facing in.

02 Slowly pull the dumbbell up towards your chest, arcing your arm back and concentrating on squeezing your back rather than letting your bicep do the work.

03 Slowly return to the start.

+

NICK'S TIP

While this is a very similar movement to a regular row, I want you to exaggerate the arcing motion so that *all* the movement is initiated from your latissimus dorsi muscle and not your biceps.

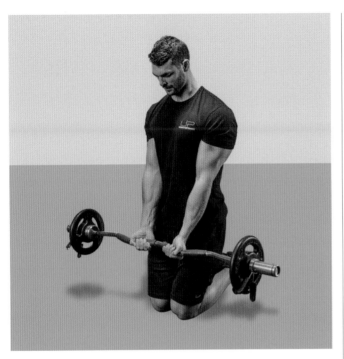

KNEELING CLOSE-GRIP EZ-BAR CURL

01 Kneel down holding an EZ-bar in front of you with a narrow underhand grip.

02 Keeping your elbows by your sides, curl the bar up towards your chin.

03 Slowly return to the start.

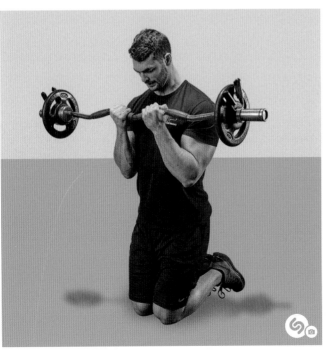

+

NICK'S TIP

You're kneeling down so that the movement becomes extremely strict. Keep it that way and forget about the weight that you're lifting; instead only focus on squeezing the biceps as hard as possible and keeping the wrists slightly cocked back so that you can isolate the biceps.

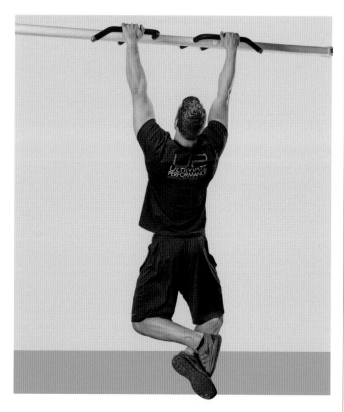

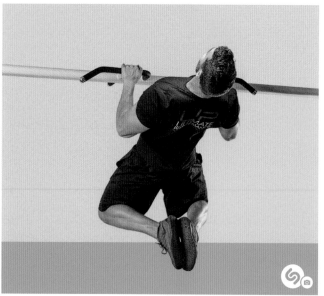

LEAN-AWAY PULL-UP

01   Hold the bar with an overhand grip with your hands shoulder-width apart.

02   Start from a dead hang with your arms fully extended and your torso leaning backwards away from the bar.

03   Pull yourself up so your chest reaches the bar by squeezing your lats.

04   Slowly return to the start.

+

NICK'S TIP

This is a tough exercise. If you find yourself struggling with it do a regular-style positive rep and then do the lean away component only on the negative portion.

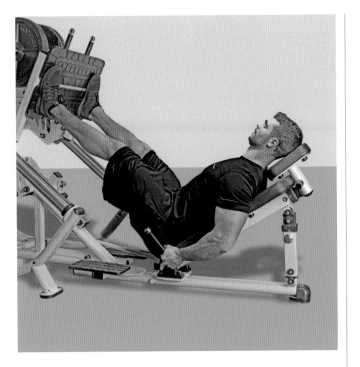

LEG PRESS

01 Sit on the machine, following its instructions to position yourself correctly and safely.

02 Release the lock, then slowly lower the platform towards you by bending your knees.

03 Push through your heels to straighten your legs and return to the start.

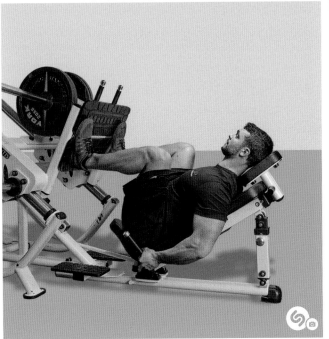

+ NICK'S TIP

Never ever lock out the knees on this exercise; 90 per cent of full leg extension is sufficient. It makes the movement safer and more effective.

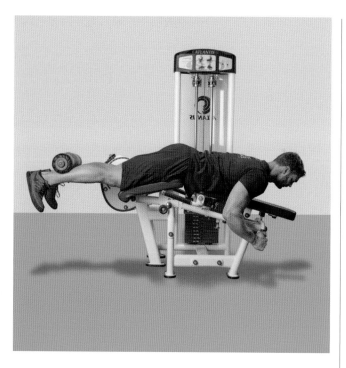

LYING HAMSTRING CURL (TOES IN*)

01 Lie on the machine, following its instructions to position yourself correctly and safely.

02 With the pad against the back of your lower calves and toes pointing inwards, raise it up by contracting your hamstrings.

03 Slowly return to the start.

* or dorsiflexed (toes up to shin)

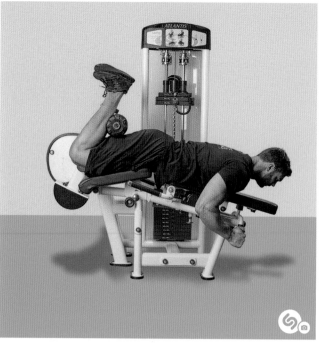

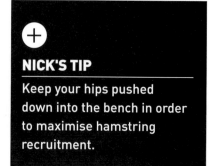

+

NICK'S TIP

Keep your hips pushed down into the bench in order to maximise hamstring recruitment.

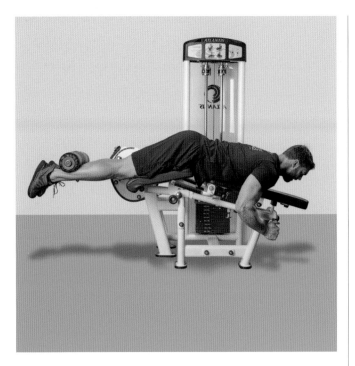

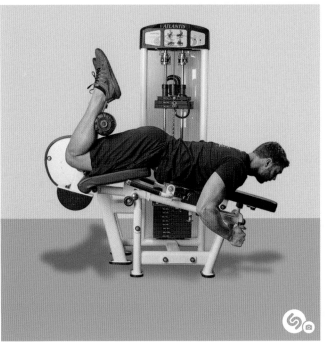

LYING HAMSTRING CURL (TOES OUT*)

01 Lie on the machine, following its instructions to position yourself correctly and safely.

02 With the pad against the back of your lower calves and toes pointing outwards, raise it up by contracting your hamstrings.

03 Slowly return to the start.

* plantar-flexed (toes away from shin)

+

NICK'S TIP

You will be weaker on this movement than with the toes-up version because it takes your calves out of the exercise. This is counterintuitive, though, as at first your calves may want to cramp simply because of how we are neurologically wired. After a workout or two this will go away as new nervous system patterns set in.

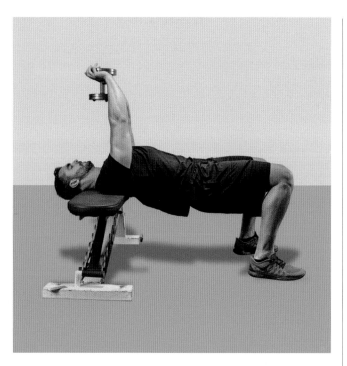

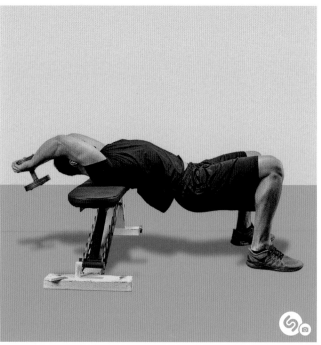

LYING SIDEWAYS DUMBBELL PULLOVER

01 Lie side on to a bench with your upper back supported with feet flat on the floor.

02 Hold a single dumbbell with both hands over your chest.

03 Slowly lower the weight behind your head, keeping a slight bend in your elbows.

04 Return the weight back to the start by raising the weight back over your ribcage with straight arms.

NICK'S TIP

Focus on keeping your shoulderblades pushed down towards your mid-back and upper arms close and tight to your body. Aim to initiate this movement using your upper back rather than pulling through the chest and triceps.

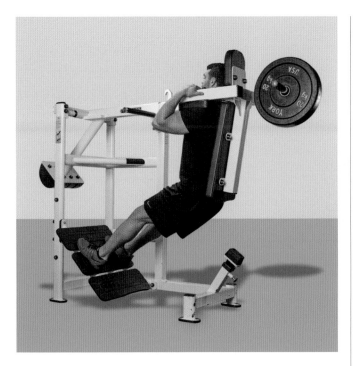

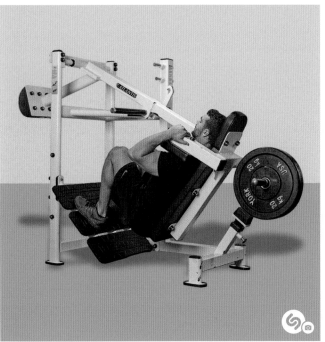

MACHINE SQUAT

01 Stand in the machine, following its instructions to position yourself correctly and safely.

02 Release the lock, then slowly bend your knees to squat down to the bottom.

03 Push through your heels to straighten your legs and return to the start.

+

NICK'S TIP

Try not to push through your toes and instead push for the outer part of the sole of your foot.

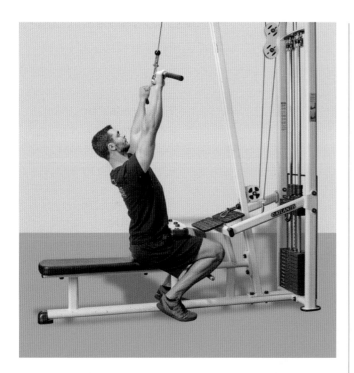

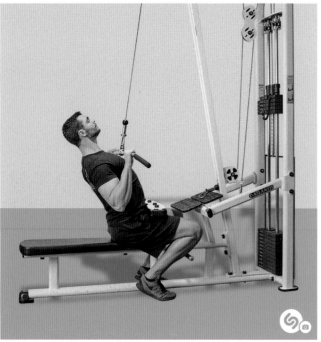

NEUTRAL SHOULDER-WIDTH LAT PULL-DOWN

01 Sit on the machine and take an overhand, shoulder-width grip on a bar attached to the high pulley cable.

02 Retract your shoulder-blades and keep your core braced.

03 Pull the bar down in front of you until it reaches your upper chest.

04 Squeeze your lats at the bottom of the move.

05 Slowly return to the start.

+ NICK'S TIP

Keep telling yourself 'chest up' at all times! You need to be able to squeeze your shoulderblades as hard as possible and you cannot do that if you are rounding your shoulders.

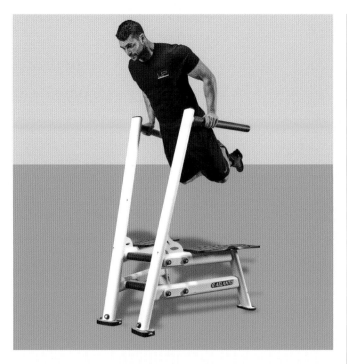

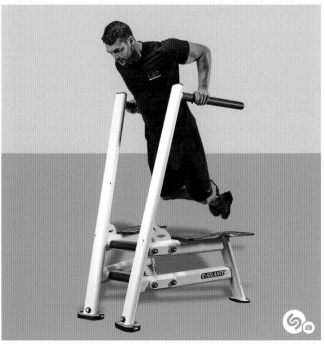

PEC DIP

01 Grip parallel bars, then lean forward as far as you can while keeping your core braced.

02 With your elbows pointing straight back, lower your body down slowly as deep as you can.

03 Press back up powerfully to return to the start.

+

NICK'S TIP

For best pectoral activation tuck your chin onto your chest and do not lock out at the top of the movement.

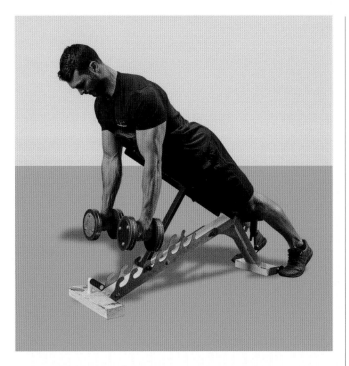

REVERSE INCLINE HAMMER CURL

01 Lie chest-first on an incline bench holding a dumbbell in each hand with palms facing.

02 Keeping your chest on the bench, curl the weights up to shoulder height.

03 Squeeze your biceps at the top of the move.

04 Slowly return to the start.

⊕

NICK'S TIP

You'll desperately want to draw your elbows back as you raise the weight. Don't do this and instead focus on keeping the upper arm pointed down perpendicular to the floor. The only time your arms can be drawn back is as you start to fatigue and want to eke out an extra rep or two, but remember that this is (good) cheating and the reps can't count towards your total!

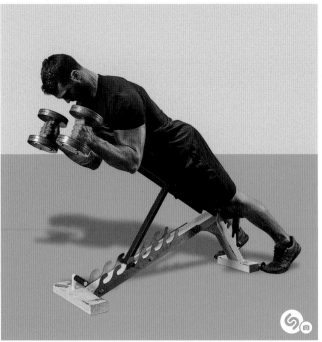

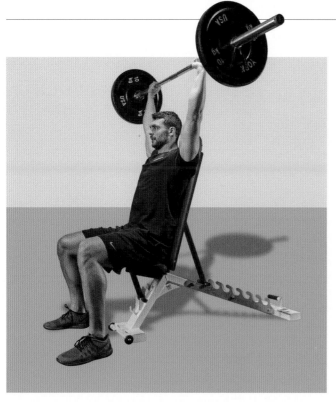

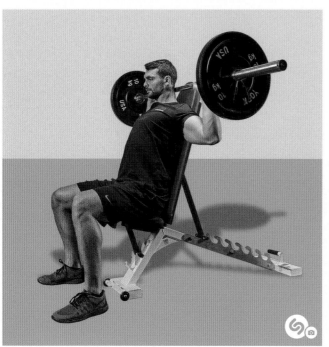

SEATED BEHIND-THE-NECK PRESS

01   Sit on an upright bench holding a bar behind your neck with a shoulder-width grip.

02   Keep your chest upright and your core muscles braced.

03   Press the bar directly upwards until your arms are straight.

04   Slowly return to the start.

✚

NICK'S TIP

Ideally you will be able to support your upper back against an upright bench on this movement. The best 'tip' here is that if you do not have the shoulder/upper chest flexibility to do this exercise in a picture-perfect fashion then switch to seated dumbbell presses.

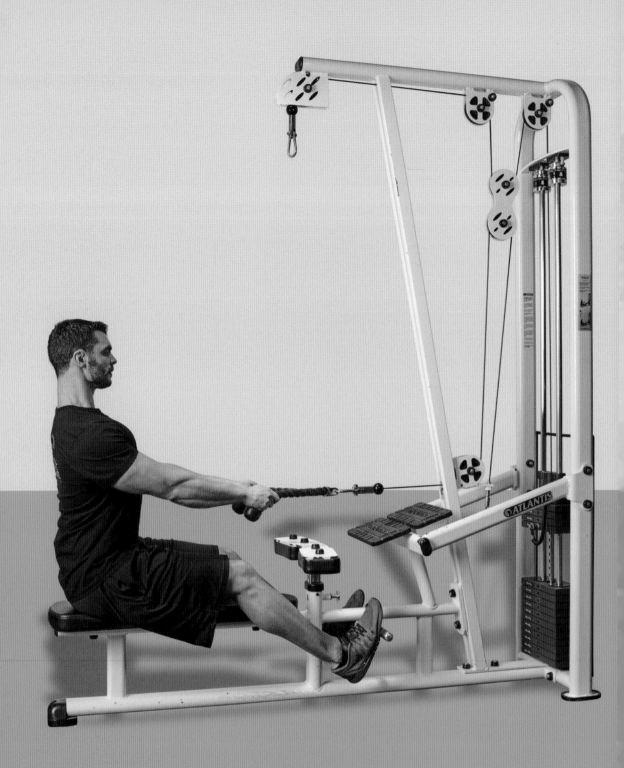

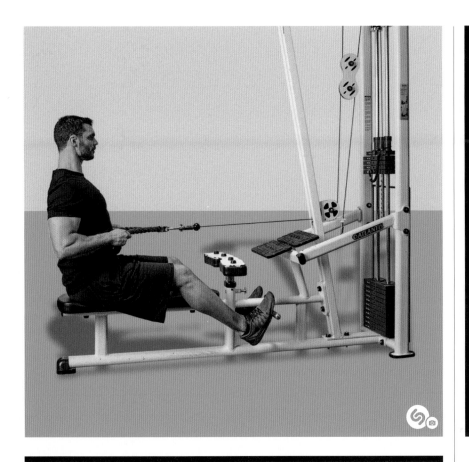

SEATED CABLE ROPE ROW

01 Sit on the machine with a slight bend in your knees, holding a double cable rope attached to the low pulley cable with an overhand grip.

02 Ensure that there is tension in the cable before you begin.

03 Pull the handle into your navel, keeping your chest up, and squeeze your shoulderblades together.

04 Slowly return to the start.

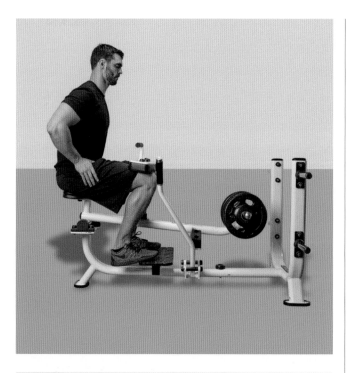

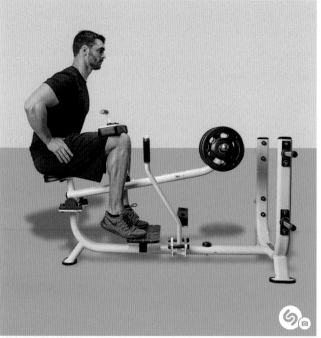

SEATED CALF RAISE

01　Sit on the machine with the pads on your quads and toes on the platform.

02　Release the safety catch and go up on to your tiptoes, keeping your chest up.

03　Slowly return to the start, ensuring your heels go below the platform for a full range of motion.

+

NICK'S TIP

Make sure you get the best possible range of motion by actively contracting your tibialis anterior (the muscle on the front of your shin) at the bottom of the movement.

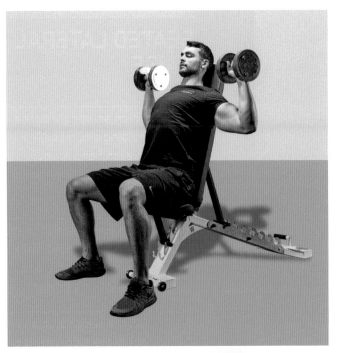

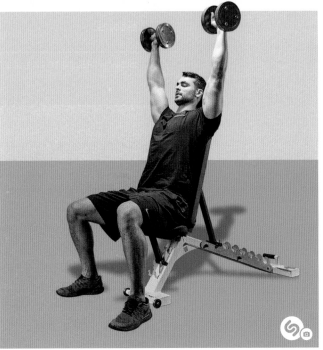

SEATED DUMBBELL SHOULDER PRESS

01 Sit on an upright bench holding a dumbbell in each hand at shoulder height with palms facing forward.

02 Keep your feet flat on the floor, core braced, back against the bench and head looking forward.

03 Press the weights up directly overhead until your arms are straight.

04 Slowly return to the start.

➕ NICK'S TIP

Don't just push the weight straight up. Instead think about contracting your deltoid muscles by keeping the elbows back and in line with the torso and ever so slightly arcing the weight up.

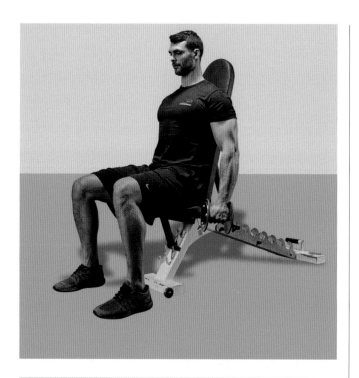

SEATED LATERAL RAISE

01 Sit on an upright bench holding a dumbbell in each hand at your sides with palms facing together.

02 Keep your feet flat on the floor, core braced, back against the bench and head looking forward.

03 Lift the weights up and out to the side, keeping a slight bend in your elbows.

04 Slowly return to the start.

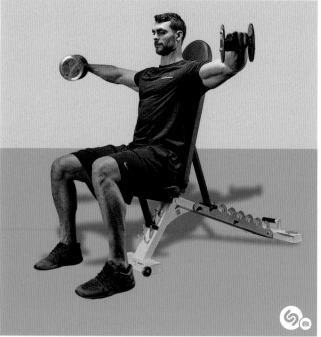

+ NICK'S TIP

Leave your ego at the door with this exercise. If it doesn't burn your medial (side) deltoids then go lighter until you can use the right muscular contraction to get the weight up. It is not about heaving, it is all about contracting.

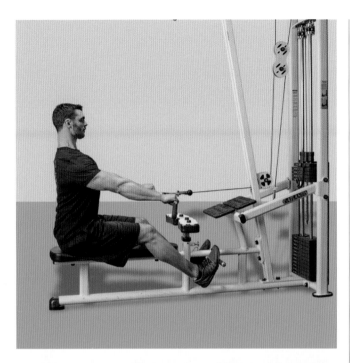

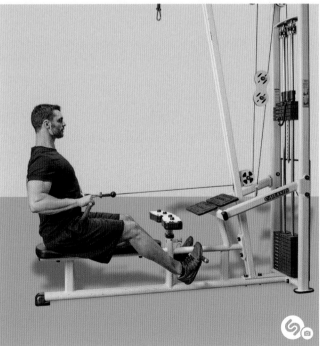

SEATED OVERHAND CABLE ROW

01 Sit on the machine with a slight bend in your knees, holding a bar attached to the low pulley cable with an overhand grip.

02 Ensure that there is tension in the cable before you begin.

03 Pull the handle into your navel, keeping your chest up, and squeeze your shoulderblades together.

04 Slowly return to the start.

⊕

NICK'S TIP

Explode on the positive part of the rep, so that you are pulling the weight into your stomach as hard as possible. Your goal should be to make the weight on the end of the cable bounce as the bar reaches your navel.

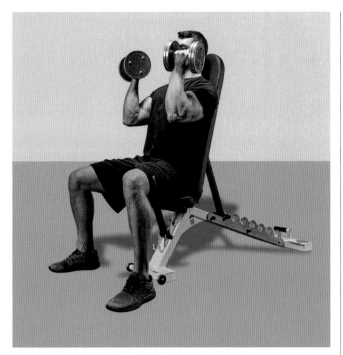

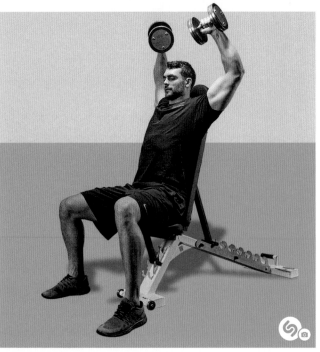

SEATED SCOTT PRESS

01   Sit on an upright bench holding a dumbbell in each hand at shoulder height with palms facing towards you.

02   Keep your feet flat on the floor, core braced, back against the bench and head looking forward.

03   Lift the weights up and out to the side, rotating your wrists so that your palms face away from you when your arms are extended.

04   Slowly return to the start.

➕ NICK'S TIP

This is an exercise where form takes extra precedence over weight. I want you to think about arcing your elbows back and up with your deltoid muscles rather than pressing the weight and using the triceps.

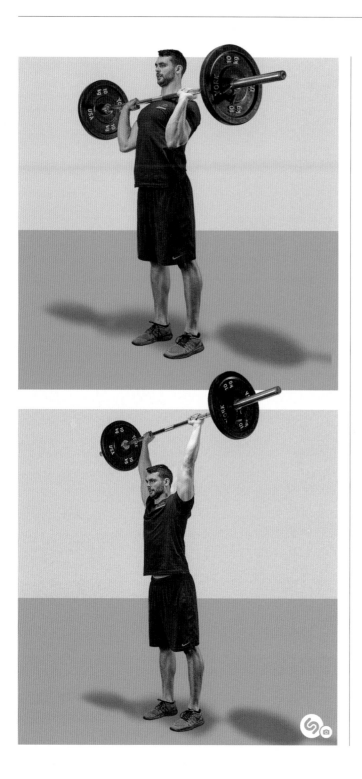

STANDING BARBELL SHOULDER PRESS

01 With your feet hip-width apart, hold a bar on your upper chest with a slightly wider than shoulder-width grip.

02 Keep your chest upright and your core muscles braced.

03 Press the bar directly upwards until your arms are straight.

04 Slowly return to the start.

➕

NICK'S TIP

For all standing upper-body exercises you can adopt a 'split stance' whereby pressure is taken off any lower back hyperextension by placing one leg anything from 2 to 20 inches in front of the rear foot.

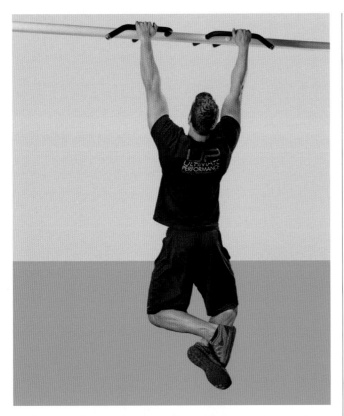

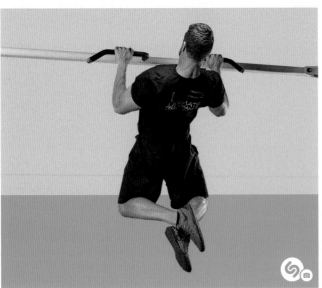

SHOULDER-WIDTH PULL-UP

01   Hold the bar with an overhand grip with your hands shoulder-width apart.

02   Start from a dead hang with your arms fully extended.

03   Pull yourself up so your chin goes over the bar by squeezing your lats.

04   Slowly return to the start.

+ NICK'S TIP

Full range of motion means all the way up and all the way down. Most gym rats need reminding of this.

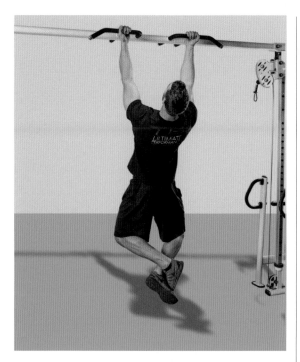

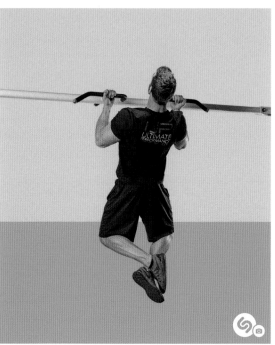

SHOULDER-WIDTH CHIN-UP

01 Hold the bar with an underhand grip with your hands shoulder-width apart.

02 Start from a dead hang with your arms fully extended.

03 Pull yourself up so your chin goes over the bar by squeezing your lats.

04 Slowly return to the start.

+

NICK'S TIP

Chin-ups should be called 'chest-ups'. Rather than the usual 'curl your chin over the bar' movement I prefer to see a 'chest to the bar' intention. You'll develop a lot more muscle and strength this way.

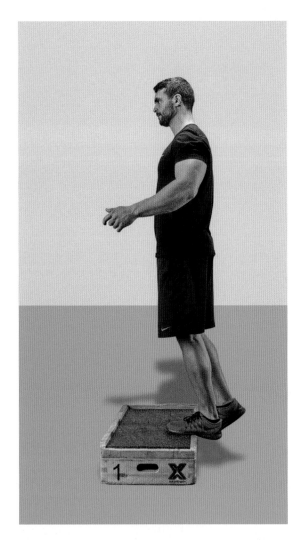
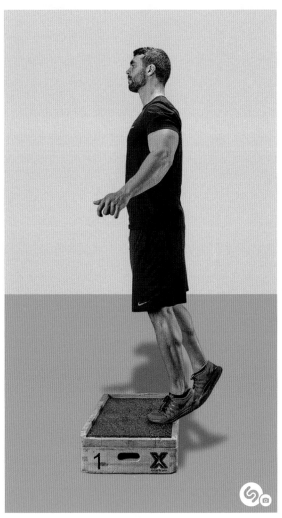

SINGLE-LEG CALF RAISE

01 Stand tall on one leg on a raised platform.

02 Go up onto your tiptoes.

03 Slowly return to the start, ensuring your heels go below the platform for a full range of motion.

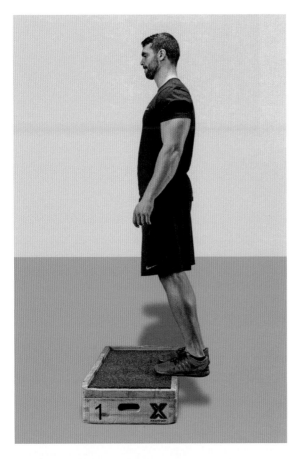

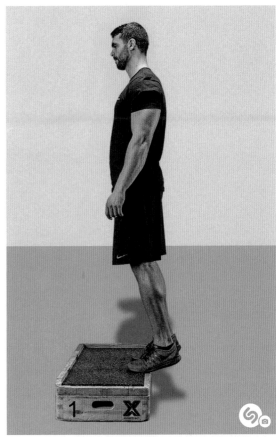

STANDING CALF RAISE

01 Stand tall on a raised platform.

02 Go up onto your tiptoes.

03 Slowly return to the start, ensuring
your heels go below the platform for a
full range of motion.

⊕ NICK'S TIP

Try these raises holding a dumbbell.
I don't mind some very small knee bend
in this movement but do resist the urge to
roll your feet – keep the weight on the ball
of your foot.

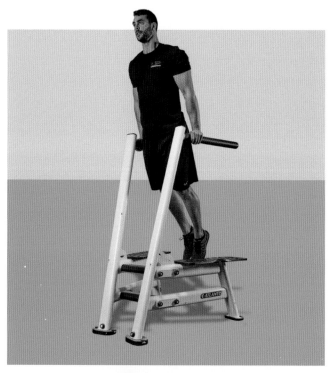

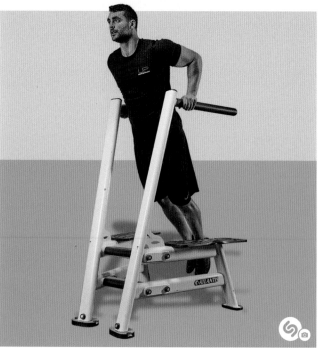

TRICEPS DIP

01 Grip parallel bars, keeping your body upright and your core braced.

02 With your elbows pointing straight back, lower your body down slowly as deep as you can.

03 Press back up powerfully to return to the start.

+

NICK'S TIP

Keep your upper body upright in order to best hit the triceps and really try to explode on the positive portion of the rep. You may not be able to actually move out of the hole all that fast, but as long as the intention is there you will recruit more triceps muscle fibres. By this stage you don't need me to also remind you that bouncing out of the bottom position is a very bad thing, do you?

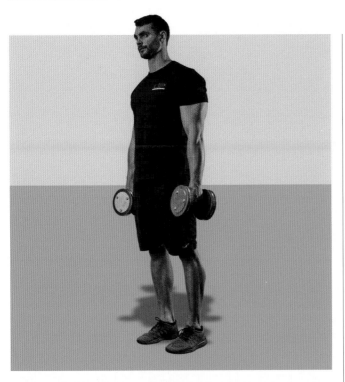

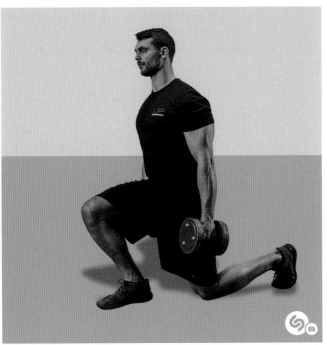

WALKING DUMBBELL LUNGES

01 Stand tall with chest up in front of a long, clear pathway, holding a dumbbell in each hand with palms facing.

02 Keeping your core braced, take a big step forward and lunge down until both knees are bent at 90°.

03 Push off from your back foot and lunge forward with that leg, and repeat.

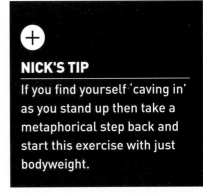

NICK'S TIP

If you find yourself 'caving in' as you stand up then take a metaphorical step back and start this exercise with just bodyweight.

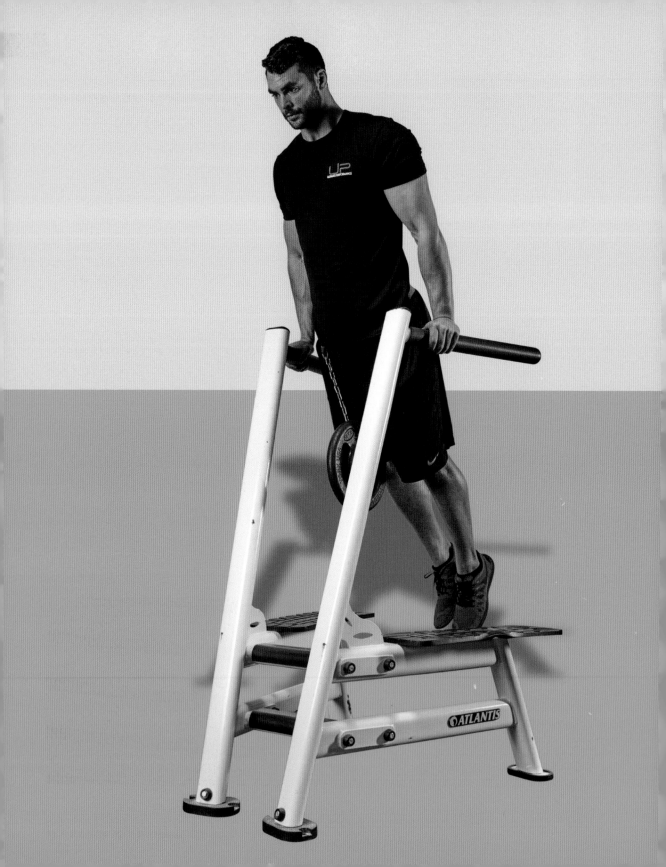

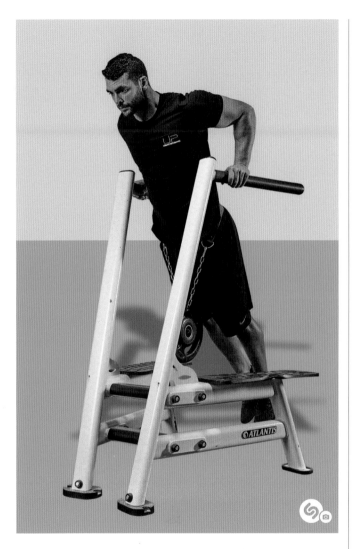

WEIGHTED TRICEPS DIP

01 Grip parallel bars, keeping your body upright and your core braced.

02 Secure a dumbbell between your feet, or use a weight plate attached to a belt.

03 With your elbows pointing straight back, lower your body down slowly as deep as you can.

04 Press back up powerfully to return to the start.

➕

NICK'S TIP

Your range should be deep enough so that you can hold a piece of paper in the fold of your elbow joint at the lowest possible part of the movement.

FOLLOWING THE PROGRAMME

YOU'RE READY TO START AND WILL NOW NEED TO CREATE YOUR OWN SPECIALLY TAILORED WORKOUT PROGRAMME BY COMBINING SPECIALISATION AND FOUNDATION WORKOUTS.

To recap, Specialisation Workouts allow you to focus on a specific area (arms, back, chest, delts, quads) over a three-week period and should be done in conjunction with the corresponding Foundation Workouts (two per week). Specialisation Workouts are numbered A to F or A to E and Foundation Workouts are numbered 1 to 36. In any week, your Foundation Workout should not cover the same area as your Specialisation Workout, so you will need to **choose only two of the three Foundation Workouts each week**

to complement your Specialisation Workout. You will drop the Foundation Workout that works the same area as the Specialisation Workout; e.g. if you choose the Arms Specialisation then drop the Arms and Delts Foundation Workout for those three weeks.

At the end of the three weeks you must choose a different Specialisation area for the next three weeks – **you should never work on the same Specialisation area in consecutive three-week periods**.

FOR EXAMPLE, IF DELTS AND CHEST ARE YOUR ONLY PRIORITIES YOU COULD FOLLOW THIS WORKOUT SPECIALISATION STRATEGY:

WEEKS 1–3 ARMS SPECIALISATION
Arms Specialisation Workouts
A to F

+

Chest and Back, Legs Foundation Workouts
1, 2, 4, 5, 7, 8 (Arms and Delts dropped
from the Foundation Workouts)

WEEKS 4–6 BACK SPECIALISATION
Back Specialisation Workouts
A to E

+

Legs, Arms and Delts Foundation Workouts
11, 12, 14, 15, 17, 18 (Chest and Back dropped
from the Foundation Workouts)

WEEKS 7–9 CHEST SPECIALISATION
Chest Specialisation Workouts
A to E

+

Legs, Arms and Delts Foundation Workouts
20, 21, 23, 24, 26, 27 (Chest and Back dropped
from the Foundation Workouts)

WEEKS 10–12 DELTS SPECIALISATION
Delts Specialisation Workouts
A to E

+

Chest and Back, Legs Foundation Workouts
28, 29, 31, 32, 34, 35 (Arms and Delts
dropped from the Foundation Workouts)

GET ON THE GRID

Use the grid on pages 150–1 to help you create your own workout routine. The grid shows all the various combinations of Specialisation and Foundation Workouts for weeks 1 to 12, with each row showing a workout session and each column showing the Specialisation area. You will only ever do one of the columns on the grid at any one time, so if you are specialising on arms, then you would only need to follow the workouts in the Arms column for three weeks. If you think of the plan as working in four lots of three-week bursts, then you will work down a column for three weeks and **you will then need to change to another Specialisation area/column** for the next 3 weeks. You can go back to the first Specialisation area after a three-week break.

The arms, back, chest and delts workout Specialisation strategy used in the example above is also shown in the annotated grid outlines on the following pages.

WEEKS 1-3
ARMS SPECIALISATION

Choose a Specialisation area and then work down that column for three weeks, alternating Specialisation and Foundation Workouts as indicated. In this case you will combine the Arms Specialisation with Chest and Back and Legs Foundation Workouts.

Letters correspond to the Specialisation Workouts you will need to do. For Arms Specialisation you will need to do Specialisation Workouts A–F.

Numbers correspond to the Foundation Workouts you will need to do. For the Arms Specialisation you will need to do Foundation Workouts 1, 2, 4, 5, 7, 8.

Use the page reference to refer back to the detailed step-by-step guide to a particular exercise.

Each workout consists of a series of exercises to be done in a set order, following the stated number of reps, sets, tempo and rest period after each set.

Moves numbered 1A and 1B, or 2A and 2B form a superset and are alternated: do all the reps of move A, rest for the stated period, then do all the reps of move B, and rest again, if a rest period is stated. Return to move A and repeat this until all the sets are done, at which point you move on to the next exercise.

Arms and Delts Foundation Workout is dropped.

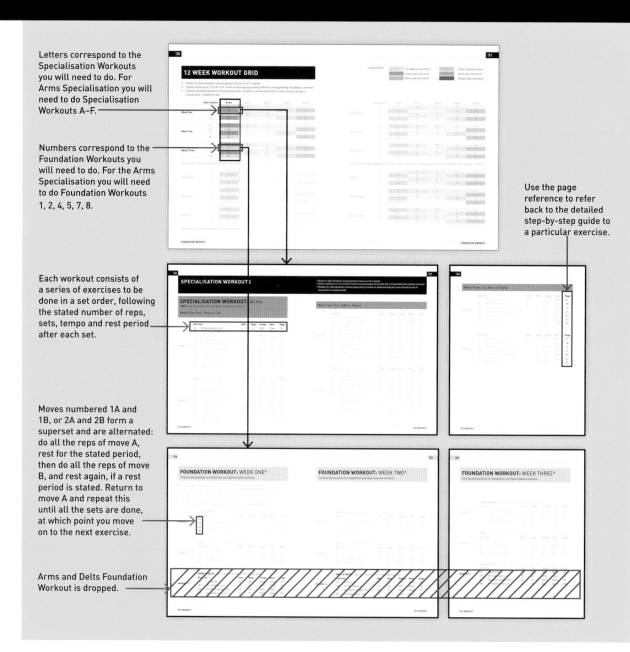

WEEKS 4-6
BACK SPECIALISATION

Choose a Specialisation area and then work down that column for three weeks, alternating Specialisation and Foundation Workouts as indicated. In this case you will combine the Back Specialisation with Legs and Arms and Delts Foundation Workouts.

Letters correspond to the Specialisation Workouts you will need to do. For Back Specialisation you will need to do Specialisation Workouts A–E.

Numbers correspond to the Foundation Workouts you will need to do. For the Back Specialisation you will need to do Foundation Workouts 11, 12, 14, 15, 17, 18.

Each workout consists of a series of exercises to be done in a set order, following the stated number of reps, sets, tempo and rest period after each set.

Use the page reference to refer back to the detailed step-by-step guide to a particular exercise.

Chest and Back Foundation Workout is dropped.

Moves numbered 1A and 1B, or 2A and 2B form a superset and are alternated: do all the reps of move A, rest for the stated period, then do all the reps of move B, and rest again, if a rest period is stated. Return to move A and repeat this until all the sets are done, at which point you move on to the next exercise.

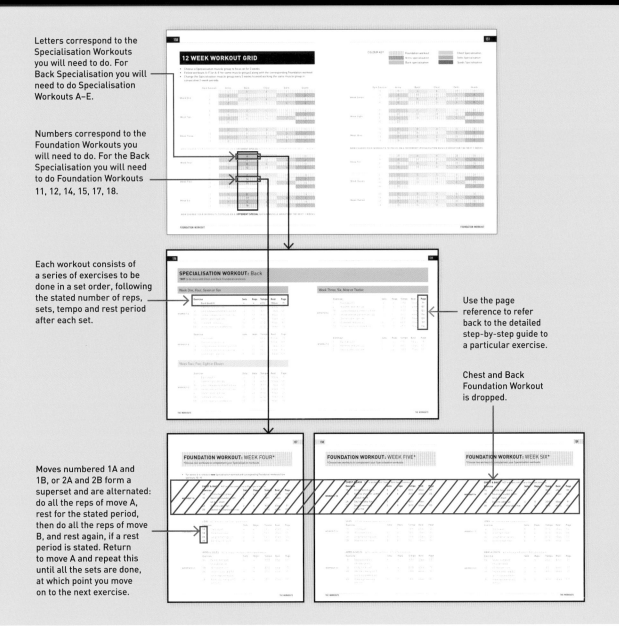

WEEKS 7-9
CHEST SPECIALISATION

Choose a Specialisation area and then work down that column for three weeks, alternating Specialisation and Foundation Workouts as indicated. In this case you will combine the Chest Specialisation with Legs and Arms and Delts Foundation Workouts.

Letters correspond to the Specialisation Workouts you will need to do. For Chest Specialisation you will need to do Specialisation Workouts A–E.

Numbers correspond to the Foundation Workouts you will need to do. For the Chest Specialisation you will need to do Foundation Workouts 20, 21, 23, 24, 26, 27.

Each workout consists of a series of exercises to be done in a set order, following the stated number of reps, sets, tempo and rest period after each set.

Use the page reference to refer back to the detailed step-by-step guide to a particular exercise.

Chest and Back Foundation Workout is dropped.

Moves numbered 1A and 1B, or 2A and 2B form a superset and are alternated: do all the reps of move A, rest for the stated period, then do all the reps of move B, and rest again, if a rest period is stated. Return to move A and repeat this until all the sets are done, at which point you move on to the next exercise.

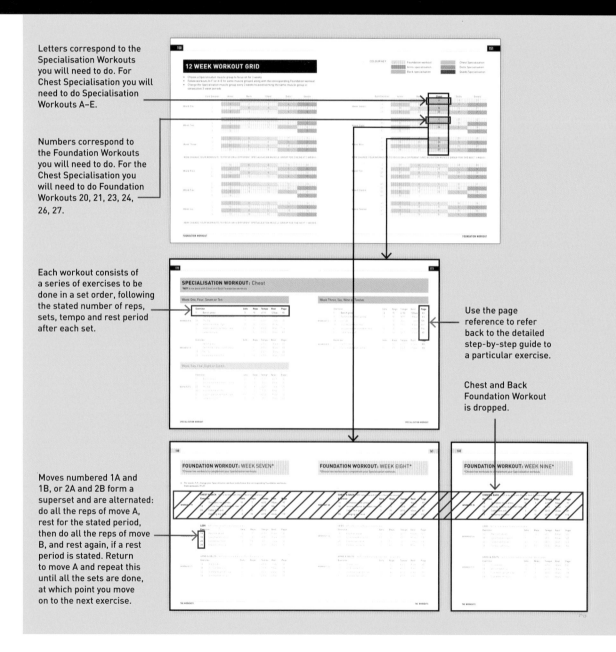

WEEKS 10-12
DELTS SPECIALISATION

Choose a Specialisation area and then work down that column for three weeks, alternating Specialisation and Foundation Workouts as indicated. In this case you will combine the Delts Specialisation with Chest and Back and Legs Foundation Workouts.

Letters correspond to the Specialisation Workouts you will need to do. For Delts Specialisation you will need to do Specialisation Workouts A–E.

Numbers correspond to the Foundation Workouts you will need to do. For the Delts Specialisation you will need to do Foundation Workouts 28, 29, 31, 32, 34, 35.

Each workout consists of a series of exercises to be done in a set order, following the stated number of reps, sets, tempo and rest period after each set.

Use the page reference to refer back to the detailed step-by-step guide to a particular exercise.

Moves numbered 1A and 1B, or 2A and 2B form a superset and are alternated: do all the reps of move A, rest for the stated period, then do all the reps of move B, and rest again, if a rest period is stated. Return to move A and repeat this until all the sets are done, at which point you move on to the next exercise.

Arms and Delts Foundation Workout is dropped.

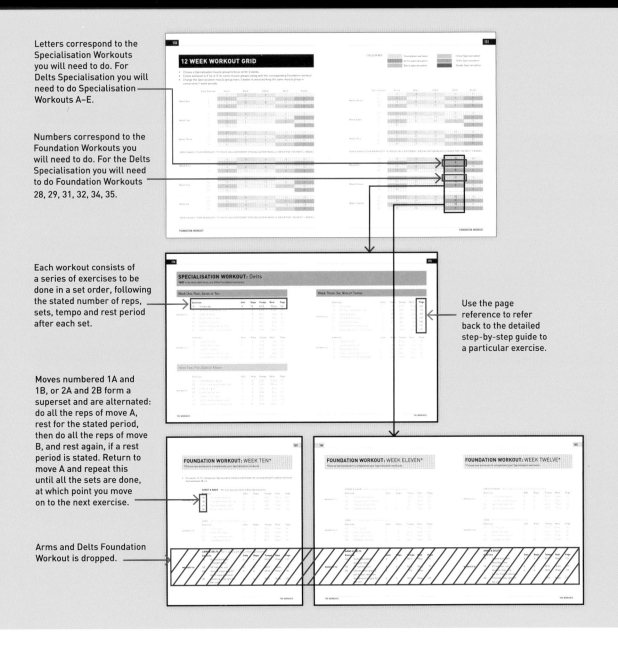

12-WEEK WORKOUT GRID

- Choose a Specialisation muscle group to focus on for 3 weeks
- Follow Workouts A–F (or A–E for some muscle groups) along with the corresponding Foundation Workout
- Change the Specialisation muscle group every 3 weeks to avoid working the same muscle group in consecutive 3-week periods

	Gym Session	Arms	Back	Chest	Delts	Quads
Week One	1	1	A	A	1	1
	2	A	2	2	A	A
	3	2	B	B	2	3
	4	B	3	3	B	B
Week Two	5	C	C	C	4	4
	6	4	5	5	5	C
	7	D	6	6	C	6
	8	5	-	-	-	D
Week Three	9	E	D	D	7	7
	10	7	8	8	D	E
	11	F	E	E	8	9
	12	8	9	9	E	F

NOW CHANGE YOUR WORKOUTS TO FOCUS ON A DIFFERENT SPECIALISATION MUSCLE GROUP FOR THE NEXT 3 WEEKS

	Gym Session	Arms	Back	Chest	Delts	Quads
Week Four	13	10	A	A	10	10
	14	A	11	11	A	A
	15	11	B	B	11	12
	16	B	12	12	B	B
Week Five	17	C	C	C	13	13
	18	13	14	14	14	C
	19	D	15	15	C	15
	20	14	-	-	-	D
Week Six	21	E	D	D	16	16
	22	16	17	17	D	E
	23	F	E	E	17	18
	24	17	18	18	E	F

NOW CHANGE YOUR WORKOUTS TO FOCUS ON A DIFFERENT SPECIALISATION MUSCLE GROUP FOR THE NEXT 3 WEEKS

COLOUR KEY

▦ Foundation Workout	▦ Chest Specialisation
▦ Arms Specialisation	▦ Delts Specialisation
▦ Back Specialisation	▦ Quads Specialisation

	Gym Session	Arms	Back	Chest	Delts	Quads
Week Seven	25	19	A	A	19	19
	26	A	20	20	A	A
	27	20	B	B	20	21
	28	B	21	21	B	B
Week Eight	29	C	C	C	22	22
	30	22	23	23	23	C
	31	D	24	24	C	24
	32	23	-	-	-	D
Week Nine	33	E	D	D	25	25
	34	25	26	26	D	E
	35	F	E	E	26	27
	36	26	27	27	E	F

NOW CHANGE YOUR WORKOUTS TO FOCUS ON A DIFFERENT SPECIALISATION MUSCLE GROUP FOR THE NEXT 3 WEEKS

	Gym Session	Arms	Back	Chest	Delts	Quads
Week Ten	37	28	A	A	28	28
	38	A	29	29	A	A
	39	29	B	B	29	30
	40	B	30	30	B	B
Week Eleven	41	C	C	C	31	31
	42	31	32	32	32	C
	43	D	33	33	C	33
	44	32	-	-	-	D
Week Twelve	45	E	D	D	34	34
	46	34	35	35	D	E
	47	F	E	E	35	36
	48	35	36	36	E	F

THE
WORKOUTS

You will find detailed step-by-step
guides to all the exercises
in the Foundation and Specialisation
Workouts in the previous section

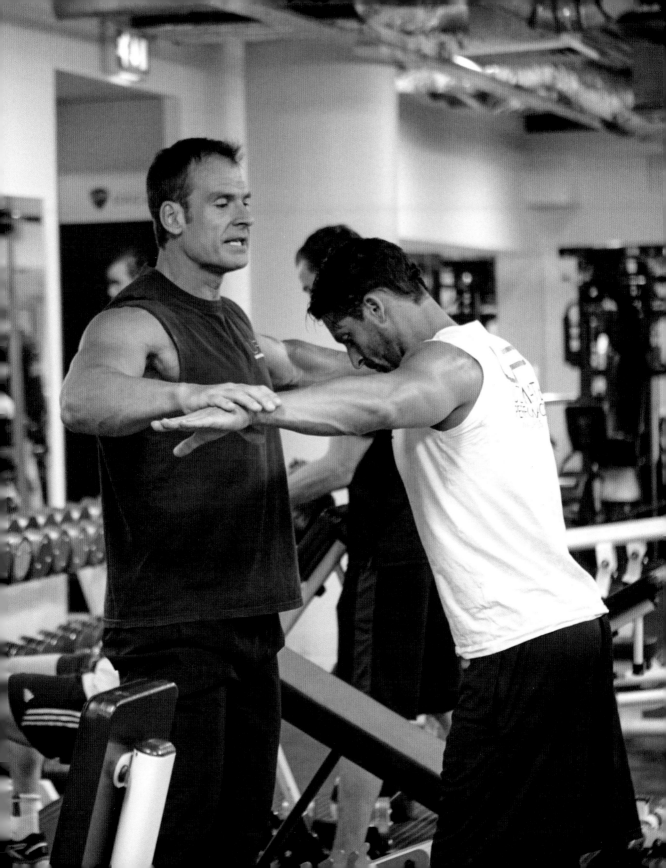

FOUNDATION WORKOUT: WEEK ONE*
*Choose two workouts to complement your Specialisation Workouts

- Your Foundation Workout should not cover the same area as your Specialisation Workout
- Over 12 weeks, follow Foundation Workouts 1–36 choosing **2 workouts each week** to complement your chosen Specialisation Workout (see pages 167–77)
- For weeks 1–3, choose your Specialisation Workout and corresponding Foundation Workouts from Workouts 1–9
- Change your Specialisation and corresponding Foundation Workouts **every 3 weeks**

WORKOUT 1

CHEST & BACK - NOT to be done with Chest or Back Specialisations

Exercise		Sets	Reps	Tempo	Rest	Page
1A	Dumbbell neck press	10	10	4010	90sec	97
1B	Incline reverse dumbbell row	10	10	4010	90sec	114
2A	Cable face pull	2	12	3011	75sec	87
2B	Incline gym ball plank	2	30	2010	60sec	113

WORKOUT 2

LEGS - NOT to be done with Quads Specialisation

Exercise		Sets	Reps	Tempo	Rest	Page
1A	Machine squat	10	10	4010	90sec	123
1B	Lying hamstring curl	10	8	4010	90sec	120
2A	Seated calf raise	2	15	3011	0sec	130
2B	Standing calf raise	2	15	2010	90sec	139

WORKOUT 3

ARMS & DELTS - NOT to be done with Arms or Delts Specialisations

Exercise		Sets	Reps	Tempo	Rest	Page
1A	Triceps dip	10	10	4010	90sec	140
1B	45° dumbbell curl	10	10	4010	90sec	76
2A	Dumbbell upright row	10	10	3010	60sec	99
2B	Dumbbell wrist curl	5	15	2010	60sec	100

FOUNDATION WORKOUT: WEEK TWO*
*Choose two workouts to complement your Specialisation Workouts

CHEST & BACK – NOT to be done with Chest or Back Specialisations

	Exercise	Sets	Reps	Tempo	Rest	Page
1A	Dumbbell neck press	10	10	4010	90sec	97
1B	Incline reverse dumbbell row	10	10	4010	90sec	114
2A	Cable face pull	3	12	3011	75sec	87
2B	Incline gym ball plank	3	20	2010	60sec	113

WORKOUT 4

LEGS – NOT to be done with Quads Specialisation

	Exercise	Sets	Reps	Tempo	Rest	Page
1A	Machine squat	10	10	4010	90sec	123
1B	Lying hamstring curl	10	8	4010	90sec	120
2A	Seated calf raise	3	15	3011	0sec	130
2B	Standing calf raise	3	15	2010	90sec	139

WORKOUT 5

ARMS & DELTS – NOT to be done with Arms or Delts Specialisations

	Exercise	Sets	Reps	Tempo	Rest	Page
1A	Triceps dip	10	10	4010	90sec	140
1B	45° dumbbell curl	10	10	4010	90sec	76
2A	Dumbbell upright row	10	10	3010	60sec	99
2B	Dumbbell wrist curl	5	15	2010	60sec	100

WORKOUT 6

FOUNDATION WORKOUT: WEEK THREE*
*Choose two workouts to complement your Specialisation Workouts

WORKOUT 7

CHEST & BACK – NOT to be done with Chest or Back Specialisations

Exercise		Sets	Reps	Tempo	Rest	Page
1A	Dumbbell neck press	10	10	4010	90sec	97
1B	Incline reverse dumbbell row	10	10	4010	90sec	114
2A	Cable face pull	4	12	3011	45sec	87
2B	Incline gym ball plank	4	20	3010	45sec	113

WORKOUT 8

LEGS – NOT to be done with Quads Specialisation

Exercise		Sets	Reps	Tempo	Rest	Page
1A	Machine squat	10	10	4010	90sec	123
1B	Lying hamstring curl	10	8	4010	90sec	120
2A	Seated calf raise	4	25	3011	0sec	130
2B	Standing calf raise	4	15	2010	90sec	139

WORKOUT 9

ARMS & DELTS – NOT to be done with Arms or Delts Specialisations

Exercise		Sets	Reps	Tempo	Rest	Page
1A	Triceps dip	10	10	4010	90sec	140
1B	45° dumbbell curl	10	10	4010	90sec	76
2A	Dumbbell upright row	10	10	3010	60sec	99
2B	Dumbbell wrist curl	5	15	2010	60sec	100

FOUNDATION WORKOUT: WEEK FOUR*
*Choose two workouts to complement your Specialisation Workouts

- For weeks 4–6, choose a **new** Specialisation Workout and corresponding Foundation Workouts from Workouts 10–18

CHEST & BACK – NOT to be done with Chest or Back Specialisations

	Exercise		Sets	Reps	Tempo	Rest	Page
WORKOUT 10	1A	Incline bench press	6	6	3010	45sec	109
	1B	Neutral shoulder-width lat pull-down	6	6	3011	45sec	124
	2A	Decline cable flye	2	8	3010	60sec	91
	2B	Seated overhand cable row	2	8	3010	60sec	133

LEGS – NOT to be done with Quads Specialisation

	Exercise		Sets	Reps	Tempo	Rest	Page
WORKOUT 11	1A	Front squat	6	6	3010	45sec	104
	1B	Glute-ham raise	6	4	3010	45sec	105
	2A	Lying hamstring curl	2	6	3010	60sec	120
	2B	Standing calf raise	2	8	3021	60sec	139

ARMS & DELTS – NOT to be done with Arms or Delts Specialisations

	Exercise		Sets	Reps	Tempo	Rest	Page
WORKOUT 12	1A	Seated dumbbell shoulder press	6	6	3010	45sec	131
	1B	60° hammer curl	6	6	3010	45sec	77
	2A	Decline close-grip EZ-bar triceps extension	6	6	3010	45sec	92
	2B	Kneeling close-grip EZ-bar curl	6	6	3010	45sec	117

FOUNDATION WORKOUT: WEEK FIVE*
*Choose two workouts to complement your Specialisation Workouts

WORKOUT 13

CHEST & BACK – NOT to be done with Chest or Back Specialisations

Exercise		Sets	Reps	Tempo	Rest	Page
1A	Incline bench press	6	6	3010	45sec	109
1B	Neutral shoulder-width lat pull-down	6	6	3011	45sec	124
2A	Decline cable flye	3	8	3010	60sec	91
2B	Seated overhand cable row	3	8	3010	60sec	133

WORKOUT 14

LEGS – NOT to be done with Quads Specialisation

Exercise		Sets	Reps	Tempo	Rest	Page
1A	Front squat	6	6	3010	45sec	104
1B	Glute-ham raise	6	4	3010	45sec	105
2A	Lying hamstring curl	3	6	3010	60sec	120
2B	Standing calf raise	3	8	3021	60sec	139

WORKOUT 15

ARMS & DELTS – NOT to be done with Arms or Delts Specialisations

Exercise		Sets	Reps	Tempo	Rest	Page
1A	Seated dumbbell shoulder press	6	6	3010	45sec	131
1B	60° hammer curl	6	6	3010	45sec	77
2A	Decline close-grip EZ-bar triceps extension	6	6	3010	45sec	92
2B	Kneeling close-grip bar curl	6	6	3010	45sec	117

FOUNDATION WORKOUT: WEEK SIX*
*Choose two workouts to complement your Specialisation Workouts

WORKOUT 16

CHEST & BACK – NOT to be done with Chest or Back Specialisations

Exercise		Sets	Reps	Tempo	Rest	Page
1A	Incline bench press	6	6	3010	45sec	109
1B	Neutral shoulder-width lat pull-down	6	6	3011	45sec	124
2A	Decline cable flye	4	8	3010	60sec	91
2B	Seated overhand cable row	4	8	3010	60sec	133

WORKOUT 17

LEGS – NOT to be done with Quads Specialisation

Exercise		Sets	Reps	Tempo	Rest	Page
1A	Front squat	6	6	3010	45sec	104
1B	Glute-ham raise	6	4	3010	45sec	105
2A	Lying hamstring curl	4	6	3010	60sec	120
2B	Standing calf raise	4	8	3021	60sec	139

WORKOUT 18

ARMS & DELTS – NOT to be done with Arms or Delts Specialisations

Exercise		Sets	Reps	Tempo	Rest	Page
1A	Seated dumbbell shoulder press	6	6	3010	45sec	131
1B	60° hammer curl	6	6	3010	45sec	77
2A	Decline close-grip EZ-bar triceps extension	6	6	3010	45sec	92
2B	Kneeling close-grip EZ-bar curl	6	6	3010	45sec	117

FOUNDATION WORKOUT: WEEK SEVEN*
*Choose two workouts to complement your Specialisation Workouts

- For weeks 7–9, change your Specialisation Workout and choose the corresponding Foundation Workouts from Workouts 19–27

CHEST & BACK – NOT to be done with Chest or Back Specialisations

	Exercise		Sets	Reps	Tempo	Rest	Page
WORKOUT 19	1A	Dumbbell neck press	10	7	4010	90sec	97
	1B	Incline reverse dumbbell row	10	7	4010	90sec	114
	2A	Cable face pull	2	10	3012	45sec	87
	2B	Hanging leg raise	2	10	4010	45sec	110

LEGS – NOT to be done with Quads Specialisation

	Exercise		Sets	Reps	Tempo	Rest	Page
WORKOUT 20	1A	Machine squat	10	7	4010	90sec	123
	1B	Lying hamstring curl	10	5	4010	90sec	120
	2A	Seated calf raise	2	15	3011	0sec	130
	2B	Donkey calf raise	2	15	2010	90sec	95

ARMS & DELTS – NOT to be done with Arms or Delts Specialisations

	Exercise		Sets	Reps	Tempo	Rest	Page
WORKOUT 21	1A	Triceps dip	10	7	4010	90sec	140
	1B	45° dumbbell curl	10	7	4010	90sec	76
	2A	Dumbbell upright row	10	7	3010	60sec	99
	2B	Dumbbell wrist curl	5	20	2010	60sec	100

FOUNDATION WORKOUT: WEEK EIGHT*

*Choose two workouts to complement your Specialisation Workouts

WORKOUT 22

CHEST & BACK - NOT to be done with Chest or Back Specialisations

Exercise		Sets	Reps	Tempo	Rest	Page
1A	Dumbbell neck press	10	6	4010	90sec	97
1B	Incline reverse dumbbell row	10	6	4010	90sec	114
2A	Cable face pull	3	10	3012	45sec	87
2B	Hanging leg raise	3	12	4010	45sec	110

WORKOUT 23

LEGS - NOT to be done with Quads Specialisation

Exercise		Sets	Reps	Tempo	Rest	Page
1A	Machine squat	10	6	4010	90sec	123
1B	Lying hamstring curl	10	4	4010	90sec	120
2A	Seated calf raise	3	15	3011	0sec	130
2B	Donkey calf raise	3	20	2010	90sec	95

WORKOUT 24

ARMS & DELTS - NOT to be done with Arms or Delts Specialisations

Exercise		Sets	Reps	Tempo	Rest	Page
1A	Triceps dip	10	6	4010	90sec	140
1B	45° dumbbell curl	10	6	4010	90sec	76
2A	Dumbbell upright row	10	6	3010	60sec	99
2B	Dumbbell wrist curl	5	20	2010	60sec	100

FOUNDATION WORKOUT: WEEK NINE*
*Choose two workouts to complement your Specialisation Workouts

WORKOUT 25

CHEST & BACK – NOT to be done with Chest or Back Specialisations

Exercise		Sets	Reps	Tempo	Rest	Page
1A	Dumbbell neck press	10	5	4010	90sec	97
1B	Incline reverse dumbbell row	10	5	4010	90sec	114
2A	Cable face pull	4	10	3012	45sec	87
2B	Hanging leg raise	4	15	4010	45sec	110

WORKOUT 26

LEGS – NOT to be done with Quads Specialisation

Exercise		Sets	Reps	Tempo	Rest	Page
1A	Machine squat	10	5	4010	90sec	123
1B	Lying hamstring curl	10	3	4010	90sec	120
2A	Seated calf raise	4	15	3011	0sec	130
2B	Donkey calf raise	4	25	2010	90sec	95

WORKOUT 27

ARMS & DELTS – NOT to be done with Arms or Delts Specialisations

Exercise		Sets	Reps	Tempo	Rest	Page
1A	Triceps dip	10	5	4010	90sec	140
1B	45° dumbbell curl	10	5	4010	90sec	76
2A	Dumbbell upright row	10	5	3010	60sec	99
2B	Dumbbell wrist curl	5	20	2010	60sec	100

FOUNDATION WORKOUT: WEEK TEN*
*Choose two workouts to complement your Specialisation Workouts

- For weeks 10–12, change your Specialisation Workout and choose the corresponding Foundation Workouts from Workouts 28–36

CHEST & BACK - NOT to be done with Chest or Back Specialisations

WORKOUT 28

Exercise		Sets	Reps	Tempo	Rest	Page
1A	Incline bench press	6	4	5010	90sec	109
1B	Shoulder-width chin-up	6	4	5010	90sec	137
2A	Decline dumbell flye	3	8	3010	75sec	94
2B	Barbell bent-over row	3	8	3010	75sec	80

LEGS - NOT to be done with Quads Specialisation

WORKOUT 29

Exercise		Sets	Reps	Tempo	Rest	Page
1A	Front squat	6	4	5010	90sec	104
1B	Glute-ham raise	6	2	6010	90sec	105
2A	Lying hamstring curl	2	5	5010	90sec	120
2B	Standing calf raise	2	12	3111	90sec	139

ARMS & DELTS - NOT to be done with Arms or Delts Specialisations

WORKOUT 30

Exercise		Sets	Reps	Tempo	Rest	Page
1A	Seated dumbbell shoulder press	6	4	5010	90sec	131
1B	60° hammer curl	6	4	5010	90sec	77
2A	Decline close-grip EZ-bar triceps extension	6	4	5010	90sec	92
2B	Kneeling close-grip EZ-bar curl	6	4	5010	90sec	117

FOUNDATION WORKOUT: WEEK ELEVEN*

*Choose two workouts to complement your Specialisation Workouts

CHEST & BACK – NOT to be done with Chest or Back Specialisations

WORKOUT 31

Exercise		Sets	Reps	Tempo	Rest	Page
1A	Incline bench press	6	5	5010	90sec	109
1B	Shoulder-width chin-up	6	5	5010	90sec	137
2A	Decline dumbell flye	3	8	3010	75sec	94
2B	Barbell bent-over row	3	8	3010	75sec	80

LEGS – NOT to be done with Quads Specialisation

WORKOUT 32

Exercise		Sets	Reps	Tempo	Rest	Page
1A	Front squat	6	5	5010	90sec	104
1B	Glute-ham raise	6	3	6010	90sec	105
2A	Lying hamstring curl	3	5	5010	90sec	120
2B	Standing calf raise	3	12	3111	90sec	139

ARMS & DELTS – NOT to be done with Arms or Delts Specialisations

WORKOUT 33

Exercise		Sets	Reps	Tempo	Rest	Page
1A	Seated dumbbell shoulder press	6	5	5010	90sec	131
1B	60° hammer curl	6	5	5010	90sec	77
2A	Decline close-grip EZ-bar triceps extension	6	5	5010	90sec	92
2B	Kneeling close-grip EZ-bar curl	6	5	5010	90sec	117

FOUNDATION WORKOUT: WEEK TWELVE*
*Choose two workouts to complement your Specialisation Workouts

WORKOUT 34

CHEST & BACK – NOT to be done with Chest or Back Specialisations

Exercise		Sets	Reps	Tempo	Rest	Page
1A	Incline bench press	6	6	5010	90sec	109
1B	Shoulder-width chin-up	6	6	5010	90sec	137
2A	Decline dumbell flye	4	8	3010	75sec	94
2B	Barbell bent-over row	4	8	3010	75sec	80

WORKOUT 35

LEGS – NOT to be done with Quads Specialisation

Exercise		Sets	Reps	Tempo	Rest	Page
1A	Front squat	6	6	5010	90sec	104
1B	Glute-ham raise	6	4	6010	90sec	105
2A	Lying hamstring curl	4	5	5010	90sec	120
2B	Standing calf raise	4	12	3111	90sec	139

WORKOUT 36

ARMS & DELTS – NOT to be done with Arms or Delts Specialisations

Exercise		Sets	Reps	Tempo	Rest	Page
1A	Seated dumbbell shoulder press	6	6	5010	90sec	131
1B	60° hammer curl	6	6	5010	90sec	77
2A	Decline close-grip EZ-bar triceps extension	6	6	5010	90sec	92
2B	Kneeling close-grip EZ-bar curl	6	6	5010	90sec	117

SPECIALISATION WORKOUT: ARMS*

*NOT to be done with Arms and Delts Foundation Workouts

Weeks One, Four, Seven or Ten

	Exercise		Sets	Reps	Tempo	Rest	Page
		Exercise	**Sets**	**Reps**	**Tempo**	**Rest**	**Page**
	1A	EZ-bar preacher curl	4	6	5010	90sec	101
	1B	Close-grip bench press	4	6	5010	90sec	88
	2A	45° dumbbell curl	3	10	3010	0sec	76
	2B	Incline dumbbell triceps extension	3	10	3010	0sec	112
	3A	Reverse incline hammer curl	3	12	4011	0sec	126
WORKOUT A	3B	Dumbbell skull-crusher	3	12	3010	90sec	98
	4A	Triceps dip	1	1	30sec	90sec	140
	4B	Hammer-grip chin-up	1	1	30sec	90sec	107
	5A	Dumbbell wrist curl	3	15	2010	0sec	100
	5B	Cable wrist curl	3	15	2011	0sec	85
	5C	Behind back barbell wrist curl	3	15	2011	0sec	82

	Exercise		Sets	Reps	Tempo	Rest	Page
		Exercise	**Sets**	**Reps**	**Tempo**	**Rest**	**Page**
	1A	EZ-bar preacher curl	4	5	5010	90sec	101
	1B	Close-grip bench press	4	5	5010	90sec	88
	2A	45° dumbbell curl	3	11	3010	0sec	76
	2B	Incline dumbbell triceps extension	3	11	3010	0sec	112
	3A	Reverse incline hammer curl	3	15	4011	0sec	126
WORKOUT B	3B	Dumbbell skull-crusher	3	15	3010	90sec	98
	4A	Triceps dip	1	1	40sec	90sec	140
	4B	Hammer-grip chin-up	1	1	40sec	90sec	107
	5A	Dumbbell wrist curl	3	15	2010	0sec	100
	5B	Cable wrist curl	3	15	2011	0sec	85
	5C	Behind back barbell wrist curl	3	15	2011	0sec	82

- Choose a Specialisation muscle group to focus on for 3 weeks
- Follow Workouts A–F (or A–E for some muscle groups) along with the corresponding Foundation Workouts
- Change the Specialisation muscle group every 3 weeks to avoid working the same muscle group in consecutive 3-week periods

Weeks Two, Five, Eight or Eleven

	Exercise	Sets	Reps	Tempo	Rest	Page
1A	EZ-bar preacher curl	5	5	5010	90sec	101
1B	Close-grip bench press	5	5	5010	90sec	88
2A	45° dumbbell curl	4	11	3010	0sec	76
2B	Incline dumbbell triceps extension	4	11	3010	0sec	112
3A	Reverse incline hammer curl	4	15	4011	0sec	126
3B	Dumbbell skull-crusher	4	15	3010	90sec	98
4A	Triceps dip	1	1	40sec	90sec	140
4B	Hammer-grip chin-up	1	1	40sec	90sec	107
5A	Dumbbell wrist curl	4	15	2010	0sec	100
5B	Cable wrist curl	4	15	2011	0sec	85
5C	Behind back barbell wrist curl	4	15	2011	0sec	82

WORKOUT C

	Exercise	Sets	Reps	Tempo	Rest	Page
1A	EZ-bar preacher curl	5	5	5010	90sec	101
1B	Close-grip bench press	5	5	5010	90sec	88
2A	45° dumbbell curl	4	11	3010	0sec	76
2B	Incline dumbbell triceps extension	4	11	3010	0sec	112
3A	Reverse incline hammer curl	4	15	4011	0sec	126
3B	Dumbbell skull-crusher	4	15	3010	90sec	98
4A	Triceps dip	1	1	40sec	90sec	140
4B	Hammer-grip chin-up	1	1	40sec	90sec	107
5A	Dumbbell wrist curl	4	15	2010	0sec	100
5B	Cable wrist curl	4	15	2011	0sec	85
5C	Behind back barbell wrist curl	4	15	2011	0sec	82

WORKOUT D

Weeks Three, Six, Nine or Twelve

WORKOUT E

Exercise		Sets	Reps	Tempo	Rest	Page
1A	EZ-bar preacher curl	2	6	5010	90sec	101
1B	Close-grip bench press	2	6	5010	90sec	88
2A	45° dumbbell curl	2	10	3010	90sec	76
2B	Incline dumbbell triceps extension	2	10	3010	90sec	112
3A	Reverse incline hammer curl	2	12	3010	90sec	126
3B	Triceps dip	2	10	3010	90sec	140
4	Cable wrist curl	2	15	2011	90sec	85

WORKOUT F

Exercise		Sets	Reps	Tempo	Rest	Page
1A	EZ-bar preacher curl	2	6	5010	90sec	101
1B	Close-grip bench press	2	6	5010	90sec	88
2A	45° dumbbell curl	2	10	3010	90sec	76
2B	Incline dumbbell triceps extension	2	10	3010	90sec	112
3A	Reverse incline hammer curl	2	12	3010	90sec	126
3B	Triceps dip	2	10	3010	90sec	140
4	Cable wrist curl	2	15	2011	60sec	85

Alternative Three-Week Arms Specialisation Workout

If you find the main arms workouts impossible to perform in a busy gym, here is an alternative workout that only requires an adjustable bench and two sets of dumbbells. This workout can be done 6 times to replace Workouts A-F. **Some of the below movements are variations on the moves in the step-by-step section, so please bear this in mind when following the form guides.**

Exercise		Sets	Reps	Tempo	Rest	Page
1A	60° incline dumbbell curl	3	10	3010	0	76
1B	60° incline hammer curl	3	10	3010	0	77
1C	Seated dumbbell curl	3	10	2010	0	75
1D	Reverse incline hammer curl	3	10	2011	0	126
1E	Incline dumbbell triceps extension	3	10	3010	0	112
1F	(Flat bench) dumbbell triceps extension	3	10	3010	0	112
1G	Seated overhead triceps extension (use 2 dumbbells)	3	10	3110	0	112
1H	(Flat bench) dumbbell chest press (with elbows tucked in tight to the body)	3	10	2010	180sec*	96

* No rest between sets but rest 180 secs after 1H

SPECIALISATION WORKOUT: BACK*

*NOT to be done with Chest and Back Foundation Workouts

Weeks One, Four, Seven or Ten

WORKOUT A

	Exercise	Sets	Reps	Tempo	Rest	Page
1	Band deadlift	4	6	4112	180sec	79
2	Hammer-grip chin-up	3	6	4010	120sec	107
3A	Lying sideways dumbbell pullover	3	10	3010	0sec	122
3B	Incline reverse one-arm arc row	3	10	3011	60sec	116
4	Seated cable rope row	2	24	2010	90sec	129
5A	Dumbbell neck press	10	10	4010	90sec	97
5B	Incline reverse dumbbell row	10	10	4010	90sec	114

WORKOUT B

	Exercise	Sets	Reps	Tempo	Rest	Page
1	Band deadlift	4	6	4112	180sec	79
2	Hammer-grip chin-up	3	6	4010	120sec	107
3A	Lying sideways dumbbell pullover	3	10	3010	0sec	122
3B	Incline reverse one-arm arc row	3	10	3011	60sec	116
4	Seated cable rope row	3	24	2010	90sec	129

Weeks Two, Five, Eight or Eleven

WORKOUT C

	Exercise	Sets	Reps	Tempo	Rest	Page
1	Band deadlift	4	6	4112	180sec	79
2	Hammer-grip chin-up	3	6	4010	120sec	107
3A	Lying sideways dumbbell pullover	3	10	3010	0sec	122
3B	Incline reverse one-arm arc row	3	10	3011	60sec	116
4	Seated cable rope row	3	24	2010	90sec	129
5A	Dumbbell neck press	10	10	4010	90sec	97
5B	Incline reverse dumbbell row	10	10	4010	90sec	114

Weeks Three, Six, Nine or Twelve

	Exercise		Sets	Reps	Tempo	Rest	Page
WORKOUT D	1	Band deadlift	4	6	4112	180sec	79
	2	Hammer-grip chin-up	3	6	4010	120sec	107
	3A	Lying sideways dumbbell pullover	3	10	3010	0sec	122
	3B	Incline reverse one-arm arc row	3	10	3011	60sec	116
	4	Seated cable rope row	3	24	2010	90sec	129
	5A	Dumbbell neck press	10	10	4010	90sec	97
	5B	Incline reverse dumbbell row	10	10	4010	90sec	114

	Exercise		Sets	Reps	Tempo	Rest	Page
WORKOUT E	1	Band deadlift	2	6	4112	180sec	79
	2	Hammer-grip chin-up	2	6	4010	120sec	107
	3	Seated cable rope row	2	24	2010	90sec	129

SPECIALISATION WORKOUT: CHEST*

*NOT to be done with Chest and Back Foundation Workouts

Weeks One, Four, Seven or Ten

	Exercise		Sets	Reps	Tempo	Rest	Page
		Exercise	Sets	Reps	Tempo	Rest	Page
WORKOUT A	1	Bench press	3	15	4110	120sec	83
	2	Decline dumbbell bench press	3	10	3010	90sec	93
	3A	Pec dip	2	15	2020	0sec	125
	3B	Incline dumbbell flye	2	10	3110	90sec	111
	4	Incline reverse dumbbell row	10	10	4010	90sec	114
	5	Cable face pull	2	12	3011	75sec	87

	Exercise	Sets	Reps	Tempo	Rest	Page
	1 Bench press	3	15	4110	120sec	83
WORKOUT B	2 Decline dumbbell bench press	3	10	3010	90sec	93
	3A Pec dip	3	15	2020	0sec	125
	3B Incline dumbbell flye	3	10	3110	90sec	111

Weeks Two, Five, Eight or Eleven

	Exercise	Sets	Reps	Tempo	Rest	Page
	1 Bench press	3	15	4110	120sec	83
	2 Decline dumbbell bench press	3	10	3010	90sec	93
WORKOUT C	3A Pec dip	3	15	2020	0sec	125
	3B Incline dumbbell flye	3	10	3110	90sec	111
	4 Incline reverse dumbbell row	10	10	4010	90sec	114
	5 Cable face pull	3	12	3011	75sec	87

Weeks Three, Six, Nine or Twelve

	Exercise		Sets	Reps	Tempo	Rest	Page
WORKOUT D	1	Bench press	3	15	4110	120sec	83
	2	Decline dumbbell press	3	10	3010	90sec	93
	3A	Pec dip	3	15	2020	0sec	125
	3B	Incline dumbbell flye	3	10	3110	90sec	111
	4	Incline reverse dumbbell row	10	10	4010	90sec	114
	5	Cable face pull	4	12	3011	45sec	87

	Exercise		Sets	Reps	Tempo	Rest	Page
WORKOUT E	1	Bench press	2	15	4110	120sec	83
	2	Decline dumbbell press	3	10	3010	90sec	93

SPECIALISATION WORKOUT: DELTS*
*NOT to be done with Arms and Delts Foundation Workouts

Weeks One, Four, Seven or Ten

	Exercise		Sets	Reps	Tempo	Rest	Page
WORKOUT A	1A	Triceps dip	10	10	4010	90sec	140
	1B	45° dumbbell curl	10	10	4010	90sec	76
	2A	Cable face pull	3	8	2012	0sec	87
	2B	Seated lateral raise	3	8	2020	0sec	132
	2C	Seated Scott press	3	8	2021	0sec	134
	2D	Incline reverse lateral raise	3	12	2012	0sec	115
	2E	Seated behind-the-neck press	3	20	2010	120sec	127

	Exercise		Sets	Reps	Tempo	Rest	Page
WORKOUT B	1A	Cable face pull	4	8	2012	0sec	87
	1B	Seated lateral raise	4	8	2020	0sec	132
	1C	Seated Scott press	4	8	2021	0sec	134
	1D	Incline reverse lateral raise	4	12	2012	0sec	115
	1E	Seated behind-the-neck press	4	20	2010	120sec	127

Weeks Two, Five, Eight or Eleven

	Exercise		Sets	Reps	Tempo	Rest	Page
WORKOUT C	1A	Dumbbell neck press	10	10	4010	90sec	97
	1B	Incline reverse dumbbell row	10	10	4010	90sec	114
	2A	Cable face pull	4	8	2012	0sec	87
	2B	Seated lateral raise	4	8	2020	0sec	132
	2C	Seated Scott press	4	8	2021	0sec	134
	2D	Incline reverse lateral raise	4	12	2012	0sec	115
	2E	Seated behind-the-neck press	4	20	2010	120sec	127

Weeks Three, Six, Nine or Twelve

	Exercise		Sets	Reps	Tempo	Rest	Page
WORKOUT D	1A	Triceps dip	10	10	4010	90sec	140
	1B	45° dumbbell curl	10	10	4010	90sec	76
	2A	Cable face pull	4	8	2012	0sec	87
	2B	Seated lateral raise	4	8	2020	0sec	132
	2C	Seated Scott press	4	8	2021	0sec	134
	2D	Incline reverse lateral raise	4	12	2012	0sec	115
	2E	Seated behind-the-neck press	4	20	2010	120sec	127

	Exercise		Sets	Reps	Tempo	Rest	Page
WORKOUT E	1A	Cable face pull	4	8	2012	0sec	87
	1B	Seated lateral raise	4	8	2020	0sec	132
	1C	Seated Scott press	4	8	2021	0sec	134
	1D	Incline reverse lateral raise	4	12	2012	0sec	115
	1E	Seated behind-the-neck press	4	20	2010	120sec	127

SPECIALISATION WORKOUT: QUADS*

*NOT to be done with Legs Foundation Workouts

Weeks One, Four, Seven or Ten

	Exercise		Sets	Reps	Tempo	Rest	Page
WORKOUT A	1A	Box jump	4	4	X	90sec	84
	1B	Lying hamstring curl	4	6	4011	90sec	120
	2A	Front squat	3	6	5010	30sec	104
	2B	Back squat	3	6	5010	120sec	78
	3	Leg press	1	50*	1010	0sec	119
	4	Walking dumbbell lunges	1	75sec	2010	0sec	141

	Exercise		Sets	Reps	Tempo	Rest	Page
WORKOUT B	1A	Box jump	4	4	X	90sec	84
	1B	Lying hamstring curl	4	6	4011	90sec	120
	2A	Front squat	4	6	5010	30sec	104
	2B	Back squat	4	6	5010	120sec	78
	3	Leg press	2	25, 50**	1010	0sec	119
	4	Walking dumbbell lunges	2	90sec	2010	120sec	141

Weeks Two, Five, Eight or Eleven

	Exercise		Sets	Reps	Tempo	Rest	Page
WORKOUT C	1A	Box jump	4	4	X	90sec	84
	1B	Lying hamstring curl	4	6	4011	90sec	120
	2A	Front squat	4	6	5010	30sec	104
	2B	Back squat	4	6	5010	120sec	78
	3	Leg press	2	25, 50**	1010	180sec	119
	4	Walking dumbbell lunges	3	90sec	2010	180sec	141

	Exercise	Sets	Reps	Tempo	Rest	Page
1A	Box jump	4	4	X	90sec	84
1B	Lying hamstring curl	4	6	4011	90sec	120
2A	Front squat	4	6	5010	30sec	104
2B	Back squat	4	6	5010	120sec	78
3	Leg press	2	25, 50**	1010	180sec	119
4	Walking dumbbell lunges	3	90sec	2010	180sec	141

WORKOUT D

Weeks Three, Six, Nine or Twelve

	Exercise	Sets	Reps	Tempo	Rest	Page
1A	Box jump	4	4	X	90sec	84
1B	Lying hamstring curl	4	6	4011	90sec	120
2A	Front squat	4	6	5010	30sec	104
2B	Back squat	4	6	5010	120sec	78
3	Leg press	2	25, 50**	1010	180sec	119
4	Walking dumbbell lunges	3	90sec	2010	180sec	141

WORKOUT E

	Exercise	Sets	Reps	Tempo	Rest	Page
1A	Box jump	2	4	X	90sec	84
1B	Lying hamstring curl	2	6	4011	90sec	120
2A	Front squat	2	6	5010	30sec	104
2B	Back squat	2	6	5010	120sec	78
3	Leg press	1	50*	1010	0sec	119

WORKOUT F

* 50-rep drop set
** 25-rep first set, then 50-rep drop set second set

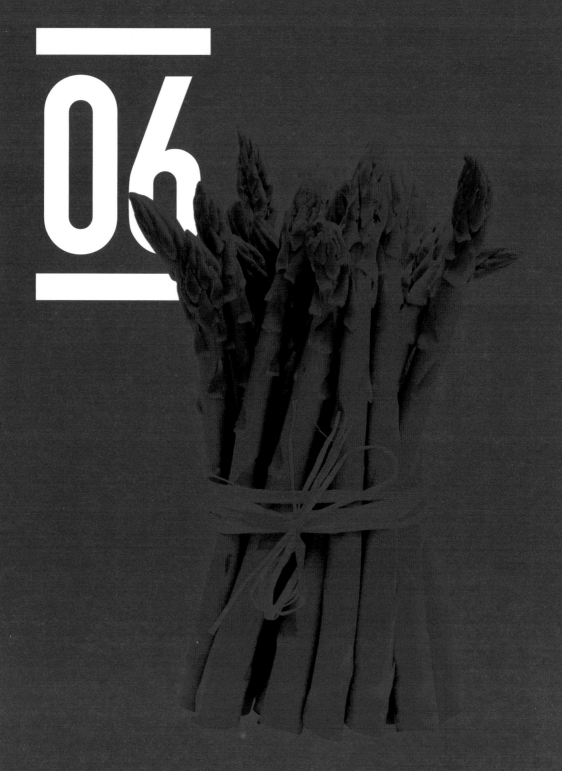

06

TRANSFORMATIONAL NUTRITION

Nowhere in the field of fitness is there more controversy and argument than on the subject of nutrition.

The information overload that comes flying at the unsuspecting newcomer is bewildering and very often not to be trusted.

The quick-fix books, the internet gurus and the pseudo-science all seem to be aimed at fleecing you rather than helping you to make informed and educated decisions.

If I can teach you just one thing to take away with you it is this: **Diet is the simplest aspect of your health and fitness regime.**

Making steady and ongoing progress from your exercise regime is always a much more complicated and intellectual affair because of the body's constant struggle with adaptation. Once you have positively adapted to an exercise stimulus you then need to change that stimulus – in a logically and structured fashion – to keep on progressing. Very rarely does the same principle hold true with diet, and for 99 per cent of your goals once you have found the way of eating that best suits you, you can stick with it and feel and look great for the rest of your life.

The problem with diet, however, is that simple and uncomplicated is not the same as 'easy'.

As challenging as the exercise programmes are in this book, they are in one way much easier to adhere to than any type of controlled diet.

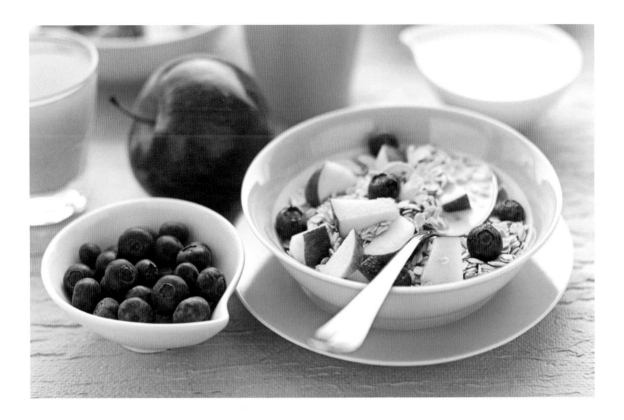

That is because four hours of exercise every week isn't an ongoing, constant thing for you to stay on top of. Controlling what you eat, on the other hand, can be a never-ending struggle against outside pressures, stress, boredom and even something as seemingly innocuous as convenience. Diet is easy to get your head around, but hard to put into practice.

I want you to keep reminding yourself of the above statement. All too often the bewildering BS of mainstream nutritional advice conflates with our own desire for shortcuts and wishful thinking (who doesn't want to eat ice cream, bacon and croissants, and get ripped and healthy at the same time?) and leads to abject confusion.

As we progress through the various approaches that you can take to your diet you will learn a variety of methodologies that have helped a huge number of 'real world' personal training clients to achieve truly stellar body composition changes. Yet the real 'diet secret' doesn't lie in the information on these pages, it lies with your desire and hunger to stick to the plan. Do not go looking to anyone else to do this for you because in the end we can all justify away any eating choice that we want.

'Just this once … one won't hurt … I'll start on Monday …' Get the excuses out of your mind if you truly want to change your body. And remember, **what you eat becomes part of you.**

THE BASIC RULES OF EATING

For the first one to two weeks adhere to this plan as strictly as possible. If you can make this diet workable for you then all by itself it will have a huge impact on your appearance and health.

BREAKFAST

You *must not* skip this meal. The ideal choice is red meat and a handful of nuts. Any cut of red meat, any type of nuts (peanuts are not nuts). If you can afford organic then opt for that. If you can't stomach red meat then eggs or oily fish are decent alternatives. Don't wait until you are in the office to eat. Aim to break your fast within 30 minutes of waking up. Beverages for breakfast: coffee and tea are fine. You can have a dash of cream in your coffee should you wish, and coconut oil is a positive addition if you like the taste. Fruit juices are off the menu.

THE REST OF THE DAY

Try to eat at least three more times, every three to five hours. And we will keep it very simple: protein and vegetables only. Going hungry leads to low blood sugar, food obsessions and dietary failure.

Protein can come from anything that has ever lived. If it has walked, crawled, slithered, flown, swam, burrowed, scampered or trotted, then you can eat it. Eggs count here as well, and dairy, if you can tolerate it, is also an option.

For the first little 'boot camp' period stick solely to green vegetables, cooked however you wish (butter is good and not to be avoided). After an initial two-week period you might add sweet potatoes or yams as options, but all vegetables are good, and don't think that a regular potato will derail your diet!

To keep it simple, at each meal you must have some animal protein and the rest must be vegetables. Eat as much as your appetite dictates; you'll be amazed how consuming the right foods leads to auto-regulation of calorie intake. The one word of caution on calorie control is to restrict nuts to breakfast only.

AFTER THE FIRST TWO WEEKS

The leaner you become the better your body can tolerate carbohydrates, and adding *complex carbohydrates* into evening meals is acceptable. The right time to consume carbs isn't in the morning as we used to believe, but in the evening to help promote restful sleep, relaxation and the right cortisol curve.

If you are really good with this diet, then a periodic break – anything from one meal to one day – every seven to 21 days can work really well. How often can you take a break and eat whatever you want? I can't answer that for you; only you can experiment and tinker to see the impact it has on your appearance, energy levels and exercise performance.

Please also note that the more frequently, and the harder, you weight train the better, because resistance training is the key exercise modality that improves insulin sensitivity and your body's ability to handle carbohydrates.

KICK-STARTING YOUR DIET, AND MAINTENANCE

How consistent and methodical you are with your diet will control the magnitude of your results.

Nothing else that you do on this programme will make as much of a difference to the way that you look and feel.

Unlike the training routines where outright novices need to start at a relatively easier level, you can jump into your diet and go straight to the advanced version. No, this does not mean that you jump straight into major calorie restriction, but you can go right to black belt methodologies from the first day. Both the eating for fat loss and eating for muscle building sections start in a logical and progressive manner so that anyone can follow them.

However, you may not want to jump in at the deep end and prefer to start slowly. Alternatively you may have worked hard to achieve your goals, made a few short-term sacrifices, and now want to ease off while maintaining your new-found physique and health.

COUNTING CALORIES

I want to have a quick word on calories. Those of you who are numbers-oriented will want to focus on calorie counting, and I am always wary of this as it can lead too many down the wrong path.

If you want to keep things simple let me assure you that calorie counting is a redundant concept for most of you. However, because there is more than one way to skin a cat, we are going to give you the tools you need if counting calories makes you feel more comfortable. But for basic, sustainable diets, do not make life more difficult than it has to be by worrying over every crumb that enters your mouth. Calories do count, but they are not all equal. Confused? If you listen to most 'experts' on this topic you will be.

All too often I encounter 'advice' from people who charge others for their advice on body composition that sets my teeth on edge. The biggest issue I have with some of these otherwise reasonably educated trainers is their total lack of grasp of what it really takes to get in great shape. It's probably wise to define what 'in great shape' actually means, because we will all have different definitions. If, and this is a big if, your goal is to get a bit slimmer, tone up, and generally look better than average but nothing special, then that is one version of being in shape and I can accept that. On the other hand, my idea of being in shape means having less than 10 per cent body fat for a man. I want the guys on my team to look special!

Achieving this level of body fat while also carrying a good degree of muscle mass is a real challenge, and something that is, to be blunt, well beyond the ken of anyone who has never done it themselves. Sure, there are some gifted guys who always hover around 8 per cent body fat come rain or shine, but these will be naturally slim, very active men with spare muscle size. So, what really gets my goat is when I read rubbish such as 'Calories don't matter so long as you only eat Paleo,' and 'I get leaner every time I increase my fat intake.' I truly despair that these unenlightened souls think it is so easy!

The fact of the matter is that when it comes to getting into real shape, the words of former world-class bodybuilder Sean Ray have resounded in my head for almost 20 years: 'Before a contest I don't go to bed a little bit hungry every night for fun.'

Bodybuilders are well known for their masochistic tendencies, and anyone who has ever got into condition to look good on stage deserves your respect for their self-discipline and persistence, but going hungry isn't something that even the iron fraternity would do out of choice. Rather it is a necessity, and the best trainers and coaches understand this, usually because they have done it themselves.

Before my words are taken too literally, I absolutely do not mean starving yourself and being permanently in famine mode! Far from it, because there are many ways to skin a cat. Some people flourish on calorie- and carb-cycling, where some days you would never know you are on a diet at all (see the meal plans section for some prime examples of how to do this). For myself, I always believe that once you carry a good degree of muscle mass and are reasonably lean, then you must have a decent amount of carbs at certain times – note the emphasis on at certain times – in order to preserve the muscle that you fought so hard to build in the first place.

But none of this individual variation can get you away from the fact that at some stage you need to create a net calorie deficit.

The reason all this misleading advice spouts forth is because the fitness industry is both extremely faddish and very often reactive, rather than proactive. For years we heard the BS that calorie counting was the only way to lose fat. This holds some truth, but the message got muddied and the so-called experts became confused. This is because the concept that 'calories count' became highjacked by low-calorie, high-sugar food manufacturers who want the unsuspecting public to believe that 200 calories from a nice bowl of low-fat, sweet-tasting cereal is actually a better breakfast for your health and appearance than 200 calories from boiled eggs.

As long as the net calories are equal all is fine, right? No, of course not. Macronutrients, among other things, have a profound impact upon hormonal and metabolic health. Only a fool would suggest otherwise.

To compound problems further, it seems that somehow the calorie debate has become mixed up with the whole carbohydrate versus fat debate. This is a cut-and-dried case of 'essential fats' being essential (wow, I hear you cry!) and, to express it as simply as possible, *fats from whole, natural foods are good for you and should not be avoided.* Excess sugar and wheat consumption, on the other hand, are major culprits in the health woes of the 21st century.

So here are the facts, and really this isn't merely my opinion, this is just the way that it is:

- Not all calories are created equal, and some are infinitely better for your body than others (think 'natural foods from the land or farm' as a general guideline here).
- Anyone who tells you calories don't count is a moron and fails to understand basic mathematics.

● To get into fantastic shape you need to educate yourself on what type of calories work best for you, and how much. It really isn't all that complicated, but it does take a bit of time to nail exactly because we are all different. Varying metabolisms, muscle mass and activity levels can change both variables massively. Sorry to disappoint you, but no book can tell you what works exactly for you; your dietary needs are too fluid for that. What this book does is lay out a range of starting maps that you need to keep working on and tinkering with.

Because I know some of you will want to know this, my own personal rule of thumb for getting into superhuman lean shape is to take in 10–12 calories per lb of bodyweight, assuming exercise levels are not crazy. That means a 200-lb man wanting to get leaner can use a calorie base of between 2,000 and 2,400 calories as a very rough starting point when working out his daily food intake.

My rough rule of thumb for gaining muscle is that a starting point for calories can be between 13 and 16 calories per lb of bodyweight, assuming you can at least see an outline of your abdominal muscles.

If truth be told I am loath to even give you this general number because the advice is just too broad and generic. The best way to work out your calorie level is to nail your maintenance diet based on the guidelines in the previous chapter, and then sit down with a pen and paper and work out how many calories you are taking in to maintain your bodyweight and keep good energy levels, all while eating a 'clean' diet.

My issue with anyone trying to calculate a calorie level prior to embarking on a correct eating regime is that the net calorie impact of 2,000 calories of standard Homer Simpson nutrition is a world away from the impact of 2,000 calories a day of The Ultimate Body Transformation Guide nutrition.

However, if it feels too much like you are winging it by not having some numbers to work towards you can base your starting diet off one of the meal plans (in this book and many more to be found in www.UltimateTransformation.Guide) and then tweak it based on your results.

NUTRITION FOR MUSCLE BUILDING

It is my sincere belief that the whole subject of nutrition and muscle building has been dramatically over-complicated by parties who have a vested interest in making things more complicated. I could easily write an entire book on the subject that would leave you confused by multiple options and no better off than if we keep it simple and to the point. To that end, this section will deal with clear rules and at the end, if you are minded to follow one, we have sample meal plans (that I loathe, but I appreciate that many of you feel the need to see one).

START AT THE BEGINNING

Most people want to kick off a new regime with all the bells and whistles possible, yet many trainers will tell you that you need to make only small incremental changes. They are partly right and partly wrong.

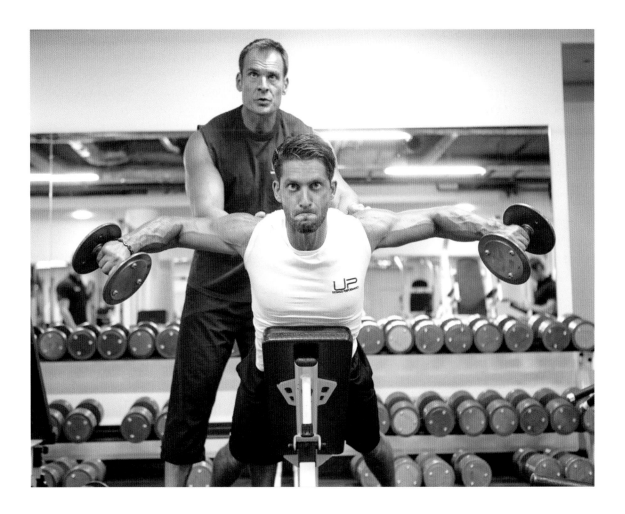

Jumping into a programme head first isn't always the worst idea, especially if you've given yourself a tight 12-week deadline, but you always need to give yourself room to tweak a plan, and you always but always need to make changes based on what you have done before. Allow me to explain further.

The very first thing we need to know when constructing your new muscle-building diet is how you have been eating previously. If you've been eating one meal a day then the initial changes we make are going to be wildly different than if you've already been eating five solid meals and downing two protein shakes every day. So the very first thing I want you to do is write down everything you've eaten for the last few days and use that as your starting point. We will get into the 'what you do next' in the rules that follow.

MOST 'HARD-GAINERS' DO NOT EAT ENOUGH FOOD

You have to eat to grow. I know it sounds a bit trite, but it is also very true, and it is arguably the number one reason for the failure of most hard-gainers' muscle-building dreams. Eating for size when you have a fast metabolism is a chore. You need to be disciplined, consistent and eat according to the clock, not according to hunger. Always stuffing your face can grow very tiresome and is the hardest part of bodybuilding for many people, skinny guys and professional bodybuilders alike.

If five meals a day are not doing the trick and everything else (training and recovery) is on point, then it is very possible that six meals a day will help accelerate progress.

WHEN IN DOUBT, EAT MORE

If muscle building is your primary transformational goal then the assumption is that you are a naturally slim and skinny individual who doesn't put fat on easily at all. If this is the case, then when in doubt always eat more. Your body is either anabolic (building up) or catabolic (breaking down), and a steady supply of calories from the right macronutrients will assist anabolism at the expense of catabolism.

This is not a prescription for the old 'bulking' staple of the 'see-food' diet – you see food and you eat it. That is wrong as too many people will end up just getting fat, which is neither healthy nor conducive to creating the right hormonal environment for muscle building. If you are full then you are full, and some of you may need to work on improving your appetite (see the supplements section for things like digestive enzymes that can help with this issue), but I don't believe in gorging and I don't believe in eating endless supplies of junk food.

NEVER SKIP A MEAL

If the rapid accumulation of muscle is your goal then I do not believe in ever skipping meals. I think that those of us who are training hard and aiming to add extra muscle tissue should eat every three hours on the clock. Apart from when sleeping!

If you read the internet forums, you may have come across the concept that meal timing is unimportant and as long as you hit your macronutrients over the course of a 24-hour period all will be fine and dandy. I hope that you can think sensibly and see that this doesn't make sense. Our hormones fluctuate during the course of the day, and so does our ability to absorb and utilise food.

When it comes to building maximum muscle what you need to understand is that your body is either synthesising protein (using amino acids to build up your body) or breaking down (cannibalising amino acids, often from your muscle tissue). There is no in-between on this. Essentially you are either anabolic or you are catabolic. Because we want to maximise anabolism we should aim to ensure that the opportunities to cannibalise muscle tissue are few and far between.

This means frequent protein feedings (research now suggests that protein synthesis peaks at about two hours after eating, which also means that non-stop grazing isn't the ideal approach if we want to maximise the peak, and returns to base levels an hour or two after that) are the order of the day. Two mega meals a day just doesn't cut it, no matter what some internet guru tells you.

The other hormonal factor that should push you towards frequent, not occasional, feedings is that stable insulin levels are important for anabolism. Small and regular feedings will help promote that.

CALORIES COUNT – SOME OF THE TIME

There is a popular notion among some modern-day trainers that 'calories don't count'. This is total BS. The law of thermodynamics applies to the human body just as it does to everything else. If we don't burn the calories we eat it must mean that the body has used them to build something. So if we need to grow we need to eat more calories than our Basal Metabolic Rate (BMR).

However, we can complicate things a little bit. Do you think that 1,000 calories from steak, baked potato and sweetcorn will have the same impact metabolically, hormonally and physiologically as 1,000 calories from bread, chocolate spread and fizzy drinks? I sincerely hope that you answered 'no'. This means that not all calories are created equal and that calorie-counting, be it for fat loss or muscle gain, only really applies when you are consistently consuming the same foods.

The way for you to approach your muscle-building diet is to keep an eye on your calorie intake (do I need to tell you that the calories must come from the 'right' foods?) and if the scale is not budging upwards in the manner that you'd like then after a five-day period boost those calories by between 5 and 15 per cent. How much you boost them is going to be down to your appetite, your fear of getting fat, whether you have boosted them before, and your ability to schedule in more or simply larger meals.

Some of you will be meticulous in tracking calories, and I have no problem at all with that. Others will be more like me and keep a rough eye on things and simply increase portion size and/or meal frequency. The absolute best way is to be precise and meticulous; after all, the better you track anything the easier it becomes to manipulate the variables needed to improve your results. But if you can't face being so precise then don't worry, it is still possible to make great gains without recording every morsel that passes your mouth.

LIQUID CALORIES VERSUS 'REAL' FOOD

A standard question that I must get asked ten times a day on Twitter is 'How many shakes can I have a day?'

No one seems to want to eat multiple meals a day and everyone looks for the shortcut provided by protein shakes. This is *wrong*.

Liquid calories can be useful at times such as post-workout, but the nutrients in 'real food' are going to promote an infinitely healthier, and therefore more responsive to muscle building, environment. However, allow me to now go on to contradict myself completely.

Whereas in an ideal world you would get your hypothetical 3,500 calories a day from five to six 'feedings' of solid food, a lot of you

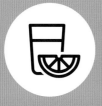

YOU CAN MAKE A CALORIE-RICH AND NUTRIENT-DENSE SHAKE OUT OF THE FOLLOWING:

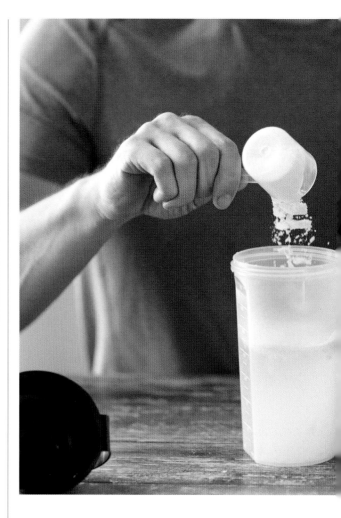

- Full-fat or raw milk. Raw milk may be difficult to purchase and if you have any concerns over its safety then you should avoid it.
- Fruit and berries. Frozen berries in a shake are great.
- Green vegetables. I know, it sounds revolting. It is. But back in the day I used to know guys who would blend up chicken breasts, so quit your whining!
- Oats.
- Flaxseed oil.
- Whey protein powder. Try to avoid the high-sugar 'weight gain powder' rubbish.
- Nuts.
- Honey.
- Yoghurt or cream. For those who really need the extra calories!

naturally skinny guys are going to really struggle to consume that quantity of food. Yes, there are tricks you can employ such as using digestive enzymes (or, even better, just eat half a papaya), but taking a person who has at best only ever eaten three smallish meals a day and asking him to jump up to six decent meals a day is often a step too far. And this is where drinking your calories can be a real blessing.

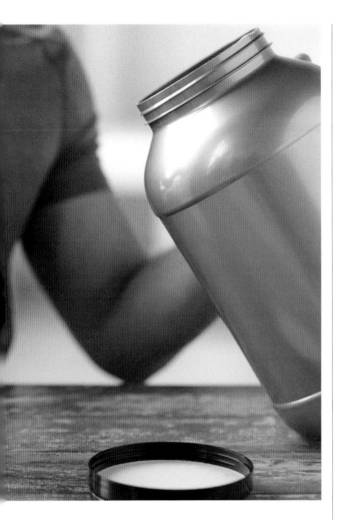

THE OVERWHELMING IMPORTANCE OF INSULIN SENSITIVITY

Understand this about the 'mother hormone' insulin:

- It is the most anabolic hormone we produce. It drives nutrients into our cells.
- For fat people it can be the devil; for skinny aspiring muscle-heads it needs to be your best friend.
- If you are lucky, your body is very insulin sensitive. This means that when you get an insulin response (typically from eating carbohydrates) your muscle cells 'open' up and take in the nutrients being shuttled by the insulin, making you bigger and more muscular.
- If you are unlucky, and most skinny guys will not have this problem as it is usually exacerbated by carrying too much body fat, you will be insulin resistant. This means that your body over-produces insulin, causing an indiscriminate shuttling of nutrients into your fat cells, making you bigger, but only because you're getting fatter, which is not the aim of the game.

For those of you who can't or won't eat solid food my advice is to make a shake (or multiple shakes, which is what I did myself when I was in my early 20s and desperate to get the biggest muscles possible) out of some or all of the following ingredients. I am not going to give you set quantities because you will all have different macronutrient and calorie goals, so you will still need to do a little bit of calculating yourself to factor this into your diet.

Now that you appreciate the importance of insulin sensitivity, the question becomes what do we do to improve or maintain it? The answer is to cycle your carbohydrate intake over the course of a few days, monitoring your body fat levels (if you start to add too much body fat then pull back on the carbs and calories for a little while), and weight train like a machine!

Two notes of warning. First, if you are carrying a spare tyre then this approach isn't for you and you need to get leaner above anything else. Second, even if you are lean, if you feel sleepy after eating a reasonable amount of carbs, such as a decent-sized serving of rice, for example, then there's a strong chance that you are naturally a bit insulin resistant. My advice if that is the case is for you to still take a carb-cycling approach, but to not be overly aggressive with higher intake days.

I am always loath to give you too many examples of how to carb cycle because what I want to teach you is the importance of listening to your body, assessing feedback (gym performance, mirror, tape measure) and adapting accordingly. It's the weakness of a book that we are forced to take a more general approach and I know it will frustrate some of you because you just want me to tell you exactly what to do.

Please understand that I cannot do this because there are so many individual factors unique to your circumstances that we need to take into account. Hence my goal is to teach you to think for yourself rather than give you overly prescriptive dogma. If you do want various real-life carb-cycle examples then please refer to the meal plans section of this book.

Carbs are 'protein sparing', which means that the more carbs you consume the less likely your body is to use carbs for its energy requirements. So while this might seem counterintuitive, whereas I might err on the high side for protein intake when on a fat-loss diet and dropping carbs, for muscle building we can keep protein a little lower than we do for certain fat-loss-focused diets.

Here is an example of how we might do things if 3,000 calories a day was your maintenance level calories and you normally ate a 40 per cent carbs (C), 30 per cent protein (P) and 30 per cent fat (F) macronutrient split. There are four calories per gram of carbs and protein and nine calories per gram of fat, so 40 per cent of your calorie intake from carbs would be 1,200 calories and 300 grams of carbs. We could, and if you want to get so detailed you should, break it down like this:

Sample macronutrient breakdown

40 per cent carbs = 1,200 cals = 300g C
30 per cent protein = 900 cals = 225g P
30 per cent fat = 900 cals = 100g F
Total calories = 3,000

If this was your hypothetical normal day's maintenance 'healthy' eating, and we decided to carb cycle for muscle gain, what's the first thing that we do?

The right answer is not to manipulate carb intake! It is to set a baseline protein goal. That's always the first nutrition rule in putting together a muscle-building diet. I like a range of 1–2g per pound of lean bodyweight. 2g is typically a bit high, if I am being honest, but we might opt for that as a goal because it's a fair strategy to get protein intake up to a decent level as hitting 1.5g out of a 2g target is much better than hitting 0.5g out of a 1g target.

If our hypothetical example weighs a lean 200lb and we are happy with his 225g of daily protein as being the minimal baseline intake, then if we carb cycle we have no wiggle room to ever drop his protein. But we can increase his protein at the expense of carbs or fat should we so desire. We can, of course, also manipulate carb and fat ratios as part of a carb-cycling approach.

CAN WE MANIPULATE CALORIE INTAKE?

Yes – but only in one direction. If 3,000 calories a day is the baseline intake to maintain current lean muscle mass then we can never go lower if optimising growth is our goal.

So now you know two things for muscle-building carb cycling:

- Baseline protein shouldn't go down. It can go up.
- Baseline calories shouldn't go down. They can go up.
- Everything else can be manipulated according to how you respond. Which is where self-experimentation comes into play.

SUPPLEMENTS CAN NEVER REPLACE FOOD

We have a specific supplements section in this book, but I want to reinforce the message that supplements are by their very definition supplementary. They are useful merely to assist a limited diet or help to push you further than normal nutrition can.

The very first thing you must do before even considering using supplements is to nail your nutrition. And if you want to get on my bad side then pop across to Twitter and tell me that you can't wait to start one of my plans but that you're not going to start until all your supplements are ready!

I am not rabidly anti or pro supplements. I think there are good and bad companies in the market and I personally take a number of products every day. We even give a couple of supplements to my young children. I am, however, very reluctant to discuss them too much because far too many people get caught up with them as a crutch. On the flip side there are also the usual nay-sayers who loathe every supplement going and throw the baby out with the bathwater.

As always, learn to think for yourself, don't buy into someone else's BS, and if a product sounds interesting for your goals then an open-minded experiment will always leave you better informed.

PROTEIN GOAL

The word 'protein' possibly derives from the Greek word 'proteios', meaning 'the first quality'. As I've already told you, working out a daily protein goal is of primary importance (the first quality) for your muscle-building efforts as we often refer to protein as being the 'building blocks' of muscle growth.

There's a lot of conjecture over the ideal protein goal for a lean adult male seeking to add muscle mass. I veer between 1g and 2g per pound of lean bodyweight, going on the high end if carbs are low and training volume is high, and coming a little bit lower if training is less frequent and carb intake is at the upper end of the scale.

To keep things extremely simple I want you to try to hit a daily target of 1.5g of protein per pound of bodyweight. So if you weigh 200lb then you should be eating 300g of protein spread out over four to six feedings.

Two quick warnings on protein intake. First, someone might try to freak you out and tell you that too much protein can damage the kidneys. Ask them to find you research where this has happened with an individual who did not already have a pre-existing kidney condition. They won't be able to find anything, no matter how hard they search.

Second, if you have a 300g protein goal, this means 300g of actual protein. It does not mean 300g of a food that is primarily protein! A lot of people go wrong in this way, because 500g of steak is 500g of steak, it is not 500g of protein. It is in fact about 100g of protein.

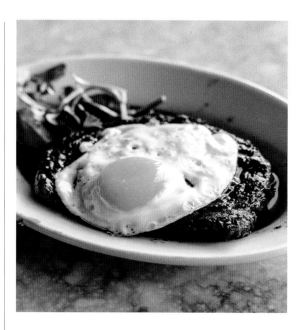

THE IMPORTANCE OF BREAKFAST

You are either anabolic (building up) or catabolic (breaking down). There is no halfway house.

After a good night's sleep the best thing for you to do is to consume some protein – the first 20g of protein you eat doesn't even go to feed your hungry muscles, it goes to support your immune system. I shouldn't need to tell you anything more because the most important message that a naturally slim person should take away from this nutritional chapter is that food is the best, and most anabolic, thing for you to focus on if you want to grow your muscles.

I'm going to add one extra bonus trick for you, though. If I was a real hard-gainer who was focusing all my efforts on maximising hypertrophy I would get up, down a quick protein shake (whey plus some essential fats), then clean my teeth and perform my daily rituals before getting down to things and cooking my breakfast.

And yes, I did write 'cooking my breakfast'. Cornflakes and a piece of toast won't cut it. The best breakfast for you is steak and eggs, with some nuts on the side. Keep the heavier carbs for later in the day when your body can better utilise them. Forget about what you may have read in the mainstream press: protein and fat will keep you alert and focused, whereas carbs will relax you.

THE IMPORTANCE OF SUPPER

Supper, the meal that you eat an hour or so before going to bed, is arguably almost as important to the aspiring muscle builder as the breakfast that we've just discussed.

Why? Because you are about to not eat for an uninterrupted period of time, so fuelling overnight muscle growth with the right foods is of critical importance. Giving you a specific supper prescription is a bit of a challenge because while some people, like myself, sleep more soundly on a full stomach, others do not. If I had to say what was more important – sleep or a full belly – I'd say sleep. That means you must pay attention to how you feel and how you sleep and adapt accordingly.

The best supper is going to be one that is more weighted towards carbs (as per the section on 'breakfast', carbs will raise insulin levels, which will in turn lower your output of the stress hormone cortisol), and raise the levels of a neurotransmitter called serotonin that is responsible for making you feel more relaxed. The end result being a more restful and sounder sleep.

There are countless supper variations that we can look at, but one great example is:

- 1 large bowl of porridge made with full-fat milk
- 2 bananas
- 4 whole eggs (any style)
- A protein shake

TWO POST-WORKOUT SHAKES

Drinking your calories can be very useful for those of you with poor appetites, but solid food is usually a better option. The one time when we should actively opt for a shake over solid food is post workout. There are arguments that a shake will be more rapidly absorbed, and I am a little on the fence with those theories, but what I will say is that a lot of us can't face a mountain of food after a hard session so shakes can be of real benefit.

One trick that I learned from world-renowned strength coach Charles Poliquin is to double up on your post-workout shake. Rather than having one big shake (for example, 50g whey, 100g carbs and 5g creatine), have two, the first (50g whey, 50g carbs and 5g creatine) immediately after a workout, and the second (30g whey and 50g carbs) an hour later.

This is a true skinny guy's trick and not for those of you who accumulate fat easily. But if it looks like you should be playing the xylophone on your ribcage then give this easy-to-follow strategy a try. It works very well indeed.

IS CHEATING GOOD?

I want you to remember what this section of the book is about. It is a relatively short-term plan designed to help you fill out certain key muscles in as short a timeframe as possible. With that caveat out of the way, allow me to introduce you to the principle of 'spike days' where we aggressively spike calories in order to further maximise growth potential and glycogen stores.

We use spike days for muscle growth in much the same way as we use carb-cycling theories. Some of you, the more precise and analytical among you, may want to stick to just carb cycling and careful tracking of everything that you eat. Others may prefer to tick along at a certain macronutrient and calorie level (above maintenance, of course, if you want to add as much muscle as possible) and then every few days (how often will depend on progress and response) have a spike day where we increase calories by up to 50 per cent.

We cannot force-feed muscle growth, but occasional high-calorie days do appear to promote extra anabolism. They are to be used judiciously and with great care. For those of you who find it pretty much impossible to ever add body fat then spike days are certainly the way to go to help you rapidly add muscular body weight.

My final point on spike days is that the first things you should eat should always be your high-quality protein. Once those are in your belly then it's time to feed the beast and eat pretty much whatever you want as long as it has some genuine nutritional value! Home-made burger and fries would be OK, ten Mars bars would not.

YOUR DIET CANNOT BE RIGID. KEEP A FOOD DIARY, ASSESS PROGRESS AND MODULATE ACCORDINGLY

I know that you want me to tell you exactly what to eat for the next 84 days. Even if I was able to squeeze all that information into a single book, I wouldn't do it because a diet needs to be a fluid and dynamic process that is a reflection of your progress, your gym performance, your ability to stay compliant, and how you are 'feeling'.

You take the starting point that we have already discussed, you start out with certain goals. At their most basic I want you to hit your protein goal but you can make it much more complicated than that if you wish. You can measure macros, calories or simply estimate portion sizes. I really am not all that concerned how you track your nutrition so long as you do follow some sort of tracking procedure. By keeping a diary you will be able to modulate your diet as you progress, taking things away or adding them depending on how your body responds. In essence this procedure allows you to learn about your own body and you become your own coach.

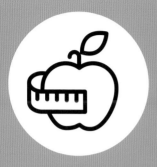

PUTTING IT ALL TOGETHER: HOW TO CONSTRUCT YOUR OWN DIET PROGRAMME

f you have read the preceding points with due care and attention you should now be in a position to put your own diet together. Remember the old saying about giving a man a fish, versus teaching him how to fish?

If you can appreciate that then you should be able to appreciate what I'm trying to do here. I want you to think for yourself so that you can construct as near as possible to your own perfect diet. Because you've probably never done this before, here are the key points:

● Establish current maintenance diet. While we should remember that all calories are not equal, they do still count. Work out what your BMR is if eating a sensible macronutrient split of 40 per cent carbs, 30 per cent protein and 30 per cent fat. That is your starting point, which you always add to.

● Break your meals down into pre- and post-workout. Unless you are training late in the day try to have more carbs post- than pre-workout.

● Harness the power of insulin. Don't skip meals and cycle carbs somewhat.

● Don't ever let yourself get hungry!

● Use liquid calories judiciously. They are not ideal but they have saved many a poor appetite.

● Do not get hooked on using supplements. Think of food as being anabolic, not a supplement pill!

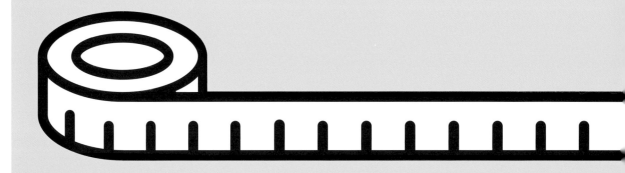

WHEN IT COMES TO EFFECTIVE FAT LOSS, IT IS VERY HARD TO OUT-TRAIN A BAD DIET

f you're a regular person who can only get to the gym four times a week for an hour at a time, then relying on your training at the expense of your diet to get rid of excess body fat means you're heading for abject failure.

Earlier in this section we discussed the concept of 'calories in, calories out', as well as giving you some commonsense guidelines on how to establish a rough calorie base. Use that information to kick-start your diet and from there please do not be afraid to experiment and keep your diet alive by playing around with calories, macronutrient ratios and even meal timings. In many ways the best diet is the diet that you stick to consistently so I do not want you to over-think things here – it is not as complicated or as bewildering as you may think.

And if you are stuck, then once you've read the following rules go to the Fat-Loss Meal Plan section and use 'Week A' as a base starter. It is full of easy ideas to get you on the right track.

RULE ONE:
GREEN IS GOOD

Make vegetables the foundation of your diet: every time you sit down to eat half your plate should be covered in a variety of green and fibrous vegetables. If you want to get lean to show off your abs then it's worth remembering that you'd have to eat half a kilo of asparagus to ingest the same amount of carbs as you get in a single wholemeal pitta bread.

RULE TWO:
EAT PROTEIN WITH EVERYTHING

Protein is one of the most important components of the diet, and when you eat a high-protein diet you're generally less hungry, eat less and lose weight as a result.

It can be a struggle to eat too much protein, although you could easily not be getting enough. Eat lean, high-quality protein with every meal and aim for a minimum of 2g per kilogram of body weight, but don't be afraid of sticking to 4g per kilo if you are in a very low-carbohydrate phase.

RULE THREE:
DON'T FEAR FAT

Fat does not make you fat. In fact, you need to consume good-quality fats if you want to build muscle and burn body fat because this macronutrient plays a number of roles in energy expenditure, vitamin storage and making testosterone, the male sex hormone. So there's no need to avoid the fats found in red meat, avocado and nuts, but avoid hydrogenated and trans fats – those found in cakes, biscuits and other processed foods – because not only will they derail your muscle-building and fat-loss mission, they are also really bad for you.

RULE FOUR:
START AS YOU MEAN TO GO ON

Think of breakfast like any other meal: you need a blend of protein, fats and veg. It may at first be strange to eat steak with broccoli first thing, but eating the right foods for breakfast will set you up for the rest of the day, get your metabolism firing and start the supply of high-quality nutrients to your muscles.

RULE FIVE:
MACRONUTRIENTS ARE MORE IMPORTANT THAN CALORIES!

What is going to make you fatter, 2,000 calories from ice cream, or 2,000 calories from steak and broccoli? You know the answer to this already, so hopefully you can accept that the intake of the correct macronutrients is ultimately more significant than mere calorie counting. Don't throw the baby out with the bathwater, as calories still do count – portion, and therefore calorie control, does have a part to play, but only once you have fixed your correct macronutrient rations, and typically only in the deeper reaches of a fat-loss programme where you are aiming to hit a low single-digit body-fat percentage.

RULE SIX:
FREE-RANGE IS PREFERABLE

Free-range animals have a more varied diet and they obtain a lot more exercise – they develop more muscle, which tends to contain more vitamins B, A and K, amino acids, iron, selenium, phosphorus and zinc. Farm-raised salmon have been found to contain up to eight times the level of carcinogens as their wild brethren, thanks to cramped conditions and poor-quality feed, while grass-fed beef tends to have much higher levels of conjugated linoleic acid and omega 3s. Eating free-range feels less like a frivolous luxury if you think of it this way: it's so nutritionally dissimilar to cage-reared that it's basically different food.

RULE SEVEN:
EAT REAL FOOD

This is the key. If you do this, you'll end up following all the other rules almost by default. A simple rule of thumb is to only eat food that grows out of the ground or food that once had a face. Alternatively, simply go caveman and think like a hunter-gatherer. When you're looking at something on the shelf, ask yourself if it would have existed 5,000 years ago. If the answer's no, it probably isn't anything that you should be eating. You may find it easier to stick to the outer aisles of the supermarket, which is where all the fresh produce is usually kept for ease of transportation, and away from the interior where everything's canned, processed or packed full of preservatives. Avoid things containing preservatives that you can't spell or ingredients you wouldn't keep in the kitchen. Eat things that will rot eventually, so that you know they're fresh. And try to enjoy it.

RULE EIGHT:
AVOID ALCOHOL

One medium-sized glass of red wine is allowed on a Saturday night. If you can factor that into your calories then there's an argument that it can be a healthy occasional addition. I don't need to tell you to avoid beer, do I?!

RULE NINE:
CARB CYCLING
FOR FAT LOSS

This can be a bewildering subject so once you've read this section please refer to the carb-cycling sections in the Fat-Loss Meal Plans for some worked-out examples of exactly how to do it.

Carbohydrates have a bad rep when it comes to muscle-building and fat loss – they spike insulin levels, which can result in your body storing more energy as fat, rather than using fat for energy – but manipulating your carb intake is one of the best ways to get bigger and leaner. You just need to be lean enough in the first place to deserve those carbs!

A WORD ON CARBS

At first glance many of the diet recommendations in this book look a lot like the dreaded Atkins Diet. This is not the case, but you will go a long way to understanding how to eat for fat loss if you can grasp that controlling your blood sugar is of pre-eminent importance. This means that carbs should only be introduced when and if your body can handle them properly.

The bad news is that if you are out of shape, you can't handle them. The good news is that weight training and getting leaner and more muscular improves insulin sensitivity. Carbs spike insulin for blood sugar management, so the better the insulin sensitivity the less indiscriminately the carbs you ingest go into fat cells and the more they go into muscle cells – where we want them to be. This means that as the 12 weeks progress you may benefit from adding carbs into your diet at some point.

After a two- to six-week low-carb period, most hard-training and strict-dieting individuals will benefit from selectively adding the right carbs into their diet. Rather than simply adding carbs on a daily basis, both science and anecdotal experience have shown that cycling your intake with low, medium and high days produces much better results for fat loss and muscle building. This way you get the muscle-building benefit of high-carb days with the fat-loss benefits of lower-carb days, all while keeping your metabolism properly revved up with fluctuating daily calorific intakes.

HOW TO DO IT

This is the most challenging part of the guide for you as the reader as it would be easy for us to tell you 'one size fits all', as you find in almost all other physique improvement books, and just follow what Joe did. But it does not work like that! You must really pay attention to your own body's feedback and adjust according to the criteria we lay out for you here.

Every five to seven days, I would tweak Joe's carb intake based on how he was performing in the gym, his overall energy levels, and his physical appearance. The right time to add carbs will come if you are eating sufficient food (if you are not, then all bets are off and you need to be more organised) and:

- You feel sluggish all the time.
- You are not getting a decent pump when you weight train, and your exercise energy levels are generally much worse than usual.
- You normally sleep well and now your sleep is disturbed.
- You are noticeably more irritable than normal.

When the time comes to add carbs to your diet, start slowly for the first five to seven days to assess how it impacts your energy and your progress, and just add 50g of carbs to your post-workout shake.

If this small addition of carbs goes well, then the next step is to add one or both of 25g extra carb powder to your post-workout shake, and a large bowl of porridge (made with water) as part of your supper at night.

This will help you sleep and get rid of those lower-carb jitters that a lot of people suffer from. Start with adding the porridge on four nights a week for the first seven days and then review. If you can't stomach porridge, you can have a medium-sized serving of wild rice, yams or sweet potatoes.

If you keep getting leaner and feel better with the addition of carbs, then one or two weeks after their gentle reintroduction is a good time to start thinking about more aggressive carb-cycling strategies. This is where it gets a bit more complicated and where estimating calories becomes a useful tool, because on the days that we add carbohydrates, if we are going for aggressive fat loss as we were with Joe, we must also take calories away via restricting either fat and/or protein intake. Before you have a heart attack and think if you reduce protein intake you will lose all that hard-earned muscle, don't worry, we'd never do that to you!

Carbs are 'protein sparing' so an increase in carbs can comfortably be accommodated by a drop in protein, especially if you have been eating close to the admittedly ambitious 4g per kilo of body weight as we have advised you to.

CARB CYCLING FOR FAT LOSS

Stick with your meat and nuts breakfast, even on high-carb days. Carbs are better post-training and later at night.

On your high-carb days only, if you want them (they are not compulsory) you can have one piece of fruit and one serving of low-fat dairy – either milk or yoghurt. The rest of your carbs should come from prescribed sources – porridge, yams, wild rice and sweet potatoes.

If you absolutely must have some bread then restrict yourself to no more than two slices of the roughest (non-processed, dark) bread. As a side note, if you find yourself a bit bloated after eating bread it's a sign that your body can't tolerate wheat and should be avoided for both aesthetic and underlying health reasons.

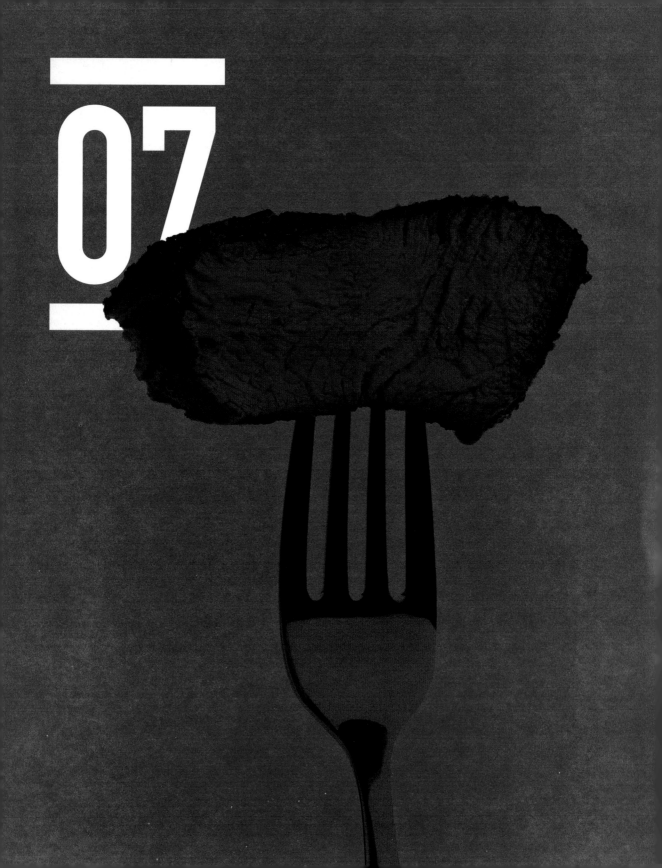

MEAL
PLANS

How to eat and
structure your
diet for muscle
building and
fat loss

If you are eating to improve your physique then we need to take into account a host of factors that will vary literally from day to day.

Let's get something straight. We cannot plan out what you should eat even two weeks in advance, let alone write a meal plan guide that you should follow to the letter. These include energy expenditure, energy requirements, digestion, performance, your response to the diet, sleeping patterns, stress levels and, unless you are a robot or a professional athlete, what is actually available to you to eat and drink on any given day.

My best response when usually asked for a generic meal plan is to tell the unsuspecting student that a sample meal plan is as useful as me giving him directions to the gym as if he was leaving from my house and not his own.

Now that I have thoroughly disillusioned you as to the validity of meal plans I'll backtrack a bit! A lot of us learn via examples – we need to see how things are laid out so that we conceptualise them ourselves. That is the overarching purpose of the muscle-building and fat-loss meal plans on the following pages. They are to give you examples of how to eat and structure your diet, and we have gone to great efforts to build on these diets in a very structured manner.

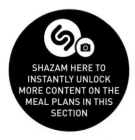

SHAZAM HERE TO INSTANTLY UNLOCK MORE CONTENT ON THE MEAL PLANS IN THIS SECTION

MUSCLE-BUILDING MEAL PLANS

I want to stress that the meal plans contained in this book are not a seamless personalised plan that runs from week 1 to week 5. They are a series of generic single-week plans that should teach you how to structure your eating. Take the time to read my explanations and then try out the approach that best fits where you are at. Various progressions have been built into the plans so in theory you could start with:

- Week A – follow for 4 weeks
- Week B – follow for 4 weeks
- Week C – follow for 2 weeks
- Week D – follow for 2 weeks

Keeping perspective

Use the layout, the structure, even the meals themselves to guide you when making your nutritional choices, but do not get hooked into portion sizes, because you will all need different amounts. Please do not raise your cortisol levels by stressing unduly about making exactly the same food choices as the examples in this book. I don't want you to think that you can't substitute a pineapple for an apple, springbok for beef, haddock for tuna, rice for potatoes. In the grand scheme of things changing between natural food choices of the same food group isn't going to make any real difference to your results.

Remember that food should be tasty and enjoyable as a huge part of dieting is sustainability. Any idiot can lose weight eating fish and cabbage, but can they keep that up? You know the answer.

To be noted:
- Vegetables were not included in macronutrient intake. Every meal was standardised to 100g green vegetables per meal.
- In some cases numbers were rounded to make things more clear.
- All macros and calorie targets were calculated through MyFitnessPal.
- In general, a fairly lean male with a relatively good response to carbohydrates was assumed.
- No supplements except BCAAs, whey protein and vitargo were used.
- All foods are readily available in supermarkets and butchers.

Abbreviations

Cho = C = Carbohydrates
Pro = P = Protein
F = Fat
Kcal = Kilocalories

MUSCLE-BUILDING PLANS: WEEK A

Macro targets: 40/30/30 split – 3,000 kcal, 300g cho/225g pro/100g fat

Training days: 4 days a week
Rationale: Kept protein and fats prior to training. Coconut oil (or MCT oils) used in pre-training meal for training energy. Carbohydrates primarily utilised post training and the two meals following to maximise post-workout anabolic window and take advantage of increased GLUT 4 translocation.

Rest days: 3 days a week
Rationale: Primarily protein and fats for first three meals in the day to help with increasing insulin sensitivity throughout the day as well as allowing increased fat oxidation. The majority of carbohydrates are in the last three meals of the day. This strategy may also help with improved drive in the earlier parts of the day. In addition, carbohydrates at night will ensure glycogen stores are full for the next day's session, especially as no carbohydrates will be consumed pre workout. The set-up can be adapted so that the first two meals are protein and fats followed by the three carbohydrate meals, before ending with protein and fats. Choosing between the two can be individual to the person. People who find they sleep well off carbohydrates can choose the former option, while those who don't can change around.

Monday

Meal plan		Macronutrient split	C	P	F
Meal 1	175g grass-fed beef fillet steak, 30g cashew nuts, 100g spinach		10	45	27
Meal 2	150g cod fillet, 25g coconut oil, 100g broccoli		0	25	26
Pre	Black coffee with 10g coconut oil		0	0	10
During	10g BCAA		0	10	0
Post	40g whey protein, 100g vitargo		100	32	2
Meal 3	140g chicken breast, 100g green beans, 110g jasmine rice,				
(1 hour later)	100g pineapple		100	40	2
Meal 4	140g chicken breast, 100g cauliflower, 110g basmati rice		85	41	3
Meal 5	140g turkey mince, 100g kale, 50g cashew butter		8	41	27
			303	234	97

Tuesday

Meal plan		Macronutrient split	C	P	F
Meal 1	150g venison mince home-made burger, 45g macadamia nuts, 100g spinach		6	40	37
Meal 2	150g line-caught haddock, 10g coconut oil, 100g broccoli		0	30	11
Pre	Black coffee with 10g coconut oil		0	0	10
During	10g BCAA		0	10	0
Post	40g whey protein, 100g vitargo		100	32	2
Meal 3	170g prawns, 100g green beans, 500g white potato, 125g red grapes		100	40	3
Meal 4	150g wild-caught tuna, 100g broccoli, 500g sweet potato		100	42	2
Meal 5	150g smoked mackerel fillets, 100g cucumber		0	32	37
			306	**226**	**102**

Wednesday

Meal plan		Macronutrient split	C	P	F
Meal 1	175g buffalo mince, 40g walnuts, 100g spinach		7	45	30
Meal 2	150g trout, 100g green beans, 20g extra virgin olive oil		3	30	30
Meal 3	150g wild-caught salmon, 100g kale, 20g grass-fed butter		0	37	22
Meal 4	140g chicken breast, 500g sweet potato, 100g broccoli		100	30	3
Meal 5	140g turkey mince, 125g basmati rice, 100g green beans		100	40	4
Pre bed	150g oatmeal, 40g casein, greens powder		90	40	15
			300	**222**	**104**

Thursday

Meal plan		Macronutrient split	C	P	F
Meal 1	150g grass-fed steak, 40g almonds, 100g spinach		8	45	32
Meal 2	150g cod fillet, 20g coconut oil, 100g broccoli		0	25	21
Pre	Black coffee with 10g coconut oil		0	0	10
During	10g BCAA		0	10	0
Post	40g whey protein, 100g vitargo		100	32	2
Meal 3	140g chicken breast, 100g green beans, 110g jasmine rice, 100g pineapple		100	40	2
Meal 4	170g jumbo king prawns, 100g runner beans, 110g basmati rice		85	40	3
Meal 5	120g turkey mince, 100g romaine lettuce, 50g cashew butter		8	37	26
			301	**229**	**96**

Friday

Meal plan		C	P	F
	Macronutrient split	**C**	**P**	**F**
Meal 1	200g grass-fed extra-lean beef mince, 30g Brazil nuts, 100g spinach	0	45	30
Meal 2	150g line-caught plaice, 10g coconut oil, 100g broccoli	0	32	23
Pre	Black coffee with 10g coconut oil	0	0	10
During	10g BCAA	0	10	0
Post	40g whey protein, 100g vitargo	100	32	2
Meal 3	175g prawns, 100g green beans, 500g white potato, 125g red grapes	100	30	2
Meal 4	150g wild-caught tuna, 100g broccoli, 500g sweet potato	100	40	2
Meal 5	150g mackerel, 100g cucumber	0	32	37
		300	**221**	**106**

Saturday

Meal plan		C	P	F
	Macronutrient split	**C**	**P**	**F**
Meal 1	3 unsmoked bacon rashers, 4 whole organic eggs, 100g spinach	4	30	28
Meal 2	175g sardines (tinned), 15g extra virgin olive oil, 100g green beans	0	38	32
Meal 3	150g wild-caught salmon, 100g kale, 20g grass-fed butter	0	37	22
Meal 4	140g chicken breast, 500g sweet potato, 100g broccoli	100	40	3
Meal 5	140g turkey mince, 125g basmati rice, 100g green beans	100	40	4
Pre bed	150g oatmeal, 40g casein, greens powder	90	45	15
		294	**230**	**104**

Sunday

Meal plan		C	P	F
	Macronutrient split	**C**	**P**	**F**
Meal 1	130g grass-fed fillet steak, 2 whole organic eggs, 100g spinach	4	30	28
Meal 2	150g mackerel, 100g green beans	0	38	32
Meal 3	150g wild-caught salmon, 100g kale	0	37	22
Meal 4	140g wild-caught tuna, 500g sweet potato, 100g broccoli	100	40	3
Meal 5	150g turkey mince burgers, 125g basmati rice, 100g green beans	100	40	4
Pre bed	150g oatmeal, 40g casein, greens powder	90	45	15
		294	**230**	**104**

MUSCLE-BUILDING PLANS: WEEK B

Macro targets: 40/30/30 split – 3,500 kcal, 350g cho/262g pro/116g fat (approx)

Training days:
Stayed the same from the first week in terms of timing and set-up, except for the increase in food in meals throughout.

Rest days:
Introduced meal 3 as a mixed meal to accommodate the increased calories in this week.

Monday

Meal plan		Macronutrient split	C	P	F
Meal 1	175g grass-fed beef fillet steak, 45g cashew nuts, 100g spinach		15	50	35
Meal 2	170g line-caught cod, 25g coconut oil, 100g broccoli		0	30	27
Pre	Black coffee with 10g coconut oil		0	0	10
During	10g BCAA		0	10	0
Post	50g whey protein, 120g vitargo		120	40	2
Meal 3	150g chicken breast, 100g green beans, 125g jasmine rice				
(1 hour later)	125g pineapple		115	45	2
Meal 4	150g chicken breast, 100g cauliflower, 125g basmati rice		100	45	3
Meal 5	150g turkey mince, 100g kale, 50g cashew butter		12	50	35
			362	270	114

Tuesday

Meal plan		Macronutrient split	C	P	F
Meal 1	190g venison home-made burger, 45g macadamia nuts, 100g spinach		8	45	40
Meal 2	220g line-caught haddock, 20g coconut oil, 100g broccoli		0	40	20
Pre	Black coffee with 10g coconut oil		0	0	10
During	10g BCAA		0	10	0
Post	50g whey protein, 120g vitargo		120	40	2
Meal 3	200g prawns, 100g green beans, 600g white potato, 125g red grapes		112	47	3
Meal 4	190g wild-caught tuna, 100g broccoli, 600g sweet potato		120	50	3
Meal 5	150g smoked mackerel fillets, 100g cucumber		0	32	37
			360	264	115

Wednesday

Meal plan		Macronutrient split	C	P	F
Meal 1	200g buffalo mince, 50g walnuts, 100g spinach		10	50	35
Meal 2	150g trout, 100g green beans, 30g extra virgin olive oil		3	35	35
Meal 3	150g wild-caught salmon, 100g kale, 20g grass-fed butter, 150g quinoa		30	45	25
Meal 4	140g chicken breast, 140g brown basmati rice, 100g broccoli		100	45	6
Meal 5	140g turkey mince, 140g basmati rice, 100g green beans		110	45	4
Pre bed	150g oatmeal, 40g casein, greens powder		90	45	13
			343	265	118

Thursday

Meal plan		Macronutrient split	C	P	F
Meal 1	175g grass-fed steak, 45g almonds, 100g spinach		9	50	37
Meal 2	170g line-caught cod, 25g coconut oil, 100g broccoli		0	30	27
Pre	Black coffee with 10g coconut oil		0	0	10
During	10g BCAA		0	10	0
Post	50g whey protein, 120g vitargo		120	40	2
Meal 3	150g chicken breast, 100g green beans, 125g jasmine rice, 125g pineapple		115	45	2
Meal 4	180g prawns, 100g runner beans, 125g basmati rice		100	45	3
Meal 5	120g turkey mince, 100g romaine lettuce, 70g cashew butter		12	42	36
			356	262	117

Friday

Meal plan	Macronutrient split	C	P	F
Meal 1	200g grass-fed extra-lean beef mince, 40g Brazil nuts, 100g spinach	0	46	35
Meal 2	200g line-caught plaice, 25g coconut oil, 100g broccoli	0	35	28
Pre	Black coffee with 10g coconut oil	0	0	10
During	10g BCAA	0	10	0
Post	50g whey protein, 120g vitargo	120	40	2
Meal 3	180g prawns, 100g green beans, 600g white potato, 125g red grapes	115	45	3
Meal 4	170g wild-caught tuna, 100g broccoli, 600g sweet potato	120	45	3
Meal 5	150g mackerel, 100g cucumber	0	32	37
		355	253	118

Saturday

Meal plan	Macronutrient split	C	P	F
Meal 1	4 unsmoked bacon rashers, 5 whole organic eggs, 100g spinach	5	40	35
Meal 2	175g sardines (tinned), 100g green beans, 22g (1.5 tbsp) extra virgin olive oil	0	40	40
Meal 3	150g wild-caught salmon, 100g kale, 20g grass-fed butter, 150g quinoa	30	45	25
Meal 4	150g chicken breast, 140g brown basmati rice, 100g broccoli	110	48	6
Meal 5	150g turkey mince, 140g basmati rice, 100g green beans	110	45	4
Pre bed	150g oatmeal, 40g casein, greens powder	90	45	13
		345	263	123

Sunday

Meal plan	Macronutrient split	C	P	F
Meal 1	130g grass-fed steak, 3 whole organic eggs, 100g spinach	6	50	37
Meal 2	150g mackerel, 100g green beans	0	32	37
Meal 3	150g wild-caught salmon, 100g kale, 20g grass-fed butter, 150g quinoa	30	45	25
Meal 4	150g wild-caught tuna, 600g sweet potato, 100g broccoli	120	45	2
Meal 5	150g turkey mince burgers, 140g basmati rice, 100g green beans	110	45	4
Pre bed	150g oatmeal, 40g casein, greens powder	90	45	10
		356	262	115

MUSCLE-BUILDING PLANS: WEEK C

Macro targets: 40/30/30 split – 3,000 kcal, 300g cho/225g pro/100g fat

Training and rest days the same as week 1, except for the following spike days:

Spike day 1 – 4,500 kcal: Ideally this would be following a high-volume workout on priority body parts to ensure muscle cells are very sensitive to the spike in nutrient intake. Two post-workout shakes would allow more nutrients to be taken in, especially considering this spike is all from 'clean' calories.

Spike day 2 – 6,000 kcal: Very large spike day, meaning it would be best carried out on a rest day, to ensure the body does not become over-stressed by both a training session and a double calorie feeding. All meals are mixed meals, including breakfast. The day ends with a 1,000 kcal free meal of choice meeting approximate macronutrient ratios of 50/25/25 (cho/pro/fat).

Monday

Meal plan	Macronutrient split	C	P	F
Meal 1	150g venison mince home-made burger, 45g macadamia nuts, 100g spinach	6	40	37
Meal 2	150g line-caught haddock, 10g coconut oil, 100g broccoli	0	30	11
Pre	Black coffee with 10g coconut oil	0	0	10
During	10g BCAA	0	10	0
Post	40g whey protein, 100g vitargo	100	32	2
Meal 3	170g prawns, 100g green beans, 500g white potato, 125g red grapes	100	40	3
Meal 4	150g wild-caught tuna, 100g broccoli, 500g sweet potato	100	42	2
Meal 5	150g smoked mackerel fillets, 100g cucumber	0	32	37
		306	226	102

Tuesday

Meal plan	Macronutrient split	C	P	F
Meal 1	175g grass-fed beef fillet steak, 65g cashew nuts, 100g spinach	20	52	42
Pre	Black coffee with 10g coconut oil	0	0	10
During	10g BCAA	0	10	0
Post 1	40g whey protein, 100g vitargo	100	32	2
Post 2	40g whey protein, 100g vitargo	100	32	2
Meal 2	120g chicken breast, 100g green beans, 110g jasmine rice, 100g pineapple	140	40	2
Meal 3	150g cod fillet, 150g basmati rice, 100g broccoli	115	40	4
Meal 4	120g chicken breast, 100g cauliflower, 110g basmati rice	115	40	4
Meal 5	120g turkey mince, 100g kale, 50g cashew butter	13	40	40
		603	**286**	**106**

Wednesday

Meal plan	Macronutrient split	C	P	F
Meal 1	175g buffalo mince, 40g walnuts, 100g spinach	7	45	30
Meal 2	150g trout, 100g green beans, 20g extra virgin olive oil	3	30	30
Meal 3	150g wild-caught salmon, 100g kale, 20g grass-fed butter	0	37	22
Meal 4	140g chicken breast, 500g sweet potato, 100g broccoli	100	30	3
Meal 5	140g turkey mince, 125g basmati rice, 100g green beans	100	40	4
Pre bed	150g oatmeal, 40g casein, greens powder	90	40	15
		300	**222**	**104**

Thursday

Meal plan	Macronutrient split	C	P	F
Meal 1	150g grass-fed steak, 40g almonds, 100g spinach	8	45	32
Meal 2	150g cod fillet, 20g coconut oil, 100g broccoli	0	25	21
Pre	Black coffee with 10g coconut oil	0	0	10
During	10g BCAA	0	10	0
Post	40g whey protein, 100g vitargo	100	32	2
Meal 3	140g chicken breast, 100g green beans, 110g jasmine rice, 100g pineapple	100	40	2
Meal 4	170g jumbo king prawns, 100g runner beans, 110g basmati rice	85	40	3
Meal 5	120g turkey mince, 100g romaine lettuce, 50g cashew butter	8	37	26
		301	**229**	**96**

Friday

Meal plan		Macronutrient split	C	P	F
Meal 1	200g grass-fed extra-lean beef mince, 30g Brazil nuts, 100g spinach		0	45	30
Meal 2	150g line-caught plaice, 10g coconut oil, 100g broccoli		0	32	23
Pre	Black coffee with 10g coconut oil		0	0	10
During	10g BCAA		0	10	0
Post	40g whey protein, vitargo		100	32	2
Meal 3	175g prawns, 100g green beans, 500g white potato, 125g red grapes		100	30	2
Meal 4	150g wild-caught tuna, 100g broccoli, 500g sweet potato		100	40	2
Meal 5	150g mackerel, 100g cucumber		0	32	37
			300	**221**	**106**

Saturday

Meal plan		Macronutrient split	C	P	F
Meal 1	150g oats, 3 large whole eggs, 40g whey protein, greens powder		90	70	30
Meal 2	200g cod fillet, 150g basmati rice, 100g avocado, 40g walnuts, 100g green beans		130	60	40
Meal 3	160g chicken breast, 150g basmati rice, 30g grass-fed butter, 100g broccoli		116	50	30
Meal 4	160g turkey lean mince, 150g jasmine rice, 100g coconut milk, 100g kale		122	50	20
Meal 5	150g oats, 100g banana, 50g raisins, 3 large eggs, 100ml liquid egg whites		150	50	30
Meal 6	Free meal		1,000 kcal at		
			50	25	25
			608	**280**	**150+**
			1,000 kcal		

Sunday

Meal plan		Macronutrient split	C	P	F
Meal 1	130g grass-fed fillet steak, 2 whole organic eggs, 100g spinach		4	30	28
Meal 2	150g mackerel, 100g green beans		0	38	32
Meal 3	150g wild-caught salmon, 100g kale		0	37	22
Meal 4	140g wild-caught tuna, 500g sweet potato, 100g broccoli		100	40	3
Meal 5	150g turkey mince burgers, 125g brown basmati rice, 100g green beans		100	40	4
Pre bed	150g oatmeal, 40g casein, greens powder		90	45	15
			294	**230**	**104**

MUSCLE BUILDING PLANS: WEEK D

Carb cycle week – 3,000 kcal approx

Ideally, the 500g carbohydrate days would fall on priority workout days, or those with the most volume, or more simply, a leg day. 250g could fall on a strength day, an upper-body day or a lesser-priority session. 50g day on a rest day after the first 500g day, with the two other rest days as 150g.

Possible splits with this cycle:

Day 1: 250g cho upper
Day 2: 500g cho lower
Day 3: 50g cho
Day 4: 250g cho upper
Day 5: 500g cho lower
Days 6 and 7: 150g cho

OR

Day 1: 250g cho upper strength
Day 2: 250g cho lower strength
Day 3: 50g cho
Day 4: 500g cho upper volume
Day 5: 500g cho lower volume
Days 6 and 7: 150g cho

Monday — 250g carbohydrates

Meal plan		Macronutrient split	C	P	F
Meal 1	175g grass-fed fillet steak, 45g almonds, 100g spinach		9	50	37
Meal 2	225g cod fillet, 20g coconut oil, 100g mange tout		0	40	22
Pre	Black coffee with 10g coconut oil		0	0	10
During	10g BCAA		0	10	0
Post	50g whey protein, 80g vitargo		80	40	3
Meal 3	160g chicken breast, 100g jasmine rice, 100g broccoli		80	44	2
Meal 4	180g prawns, 100g basmati rice, 100g runner beans		80	40	3
Meal 5	140g turkey mince home-made burgers, 50g cashew butter, 100g kale		8	40	27
			257	264	104

Tuesday   500g carbohydrates

Meal plan		Macronutrient split	C	P	F
Meal 1	120g venison mince, 10g coconut oil, 100g spinach		0	26	14
Pre	Black coffee				
During	10g BCAA		0	10	0
Post	40g whey protein, 120g vitargo		120	32	0
Meal 2	110g chicken breast, 600g white potato, 100g banana, 100g broccoli		115	35	2
Meal 3	150g cod fillet, 600g sweet potato, 100g green beans		120	35	2
Meal 4	130g haddock fillet, 100g basmati rice, 100g kale		75	30	2
Meal 5	120g venison steak, 100g basmati rice, 100g asparagus		75	35	3
			505	**203**	**23**

Wednesday   50g carbohydrates

Meal plan		Macronutrient split	C	P	F
Meal 1	200g extra-lean buffalo mince, 50g walnuts, 100g green beans		9	50	36
Meal 2	180g trout, 30g extra virgin olive oil, 100g broccoli		4	40	37
Meal 3	180g wild Alaskan salmon, 30g grass-fed butter, 100g spinach		0	45	32
Meal 4	200g turkey lean mince, 50g peanut butter, 100g asparagus		4	60	31
Meal 5	150g mackerel, 100g cucumber		0	32	37
Meal 6	200g chicken breast, 200g sweet potato, 100g kale		40	48	2
			57	**275**	**175**

Thursday   250g carbohydrates

Meal plan		Macronutrient split	C	P	F
Meal 1	175g grass-fed fillet steak, 45g almonds, 100g spinach		9	50	37
Meal 2	225g cod fillet, 20g coconut oil, 100g mange tout		0	40	22
Pre	Black coffee with 10g coconut oil		0	0	10
During	10g BCAA		0	10	0
Post	50g whey protein, 80g vitargo		80	40	3
Meal 3	160g chicken breast, 100g jasmine rice, 100g broccoli		80	44	2
Meal 4	180g prawns, 100g basmati rice, 100g runner beans		80	40	3
Meal 5	140g turkey mince home-made burgers, 50g cashew butter, 100g kale		80	40	27
			329	**264**	**104**

Friday — 500g carbohydrates

Meal plan		Macronutrient split	C	P	F
Meal 1	120g venison mince, 10g coconut oil, 100g spinach		0	26	14
Pre	Black coffee		-		
During	10g BCAA		0	10	0
Post	40g whey protein, 120g vitargo		120	32	0
Meal 2	110g chicken breast, 600g white potato, 100g banana, 100g broccoli		115	35	2
Meal 3	150g cod fillet, 600g sweet potato, 100g green beans		120	35	2
Meal 4	130g haddock fillet, 100g basmati rice, 100g kale		75	30	2
Meal 5	120g venison steak, 100g basmati rice, 100g asparagus		75	35	3
			505	203	23

Saturday — 150g carbohydrates

Meal plan		Macronutrient split	C	P	F
Meal 1	200g extra-lean buffalo mince, 40g walnuts, 100g spinach		8	50	30
Meal 2	180g trout, 25g extra virgin olive oil, 100g green beans		4	40	33
Meal 3	180g wild Alaskan salmon, 30g grass-fed butter, 100g kale		0	44	32
Meal 4	200g lean turkey mince, 50g peanut butter, 100g asparagus		4	60	30
Meal 5	225g cod fillet, 350g sweet potato, 100g Brussels sprouts		70	44	2
Meal 6	100g oats, 50g whey protein, greens powder		65	50	10
			151	288	137

Sunday — 150g carbohydrates

Meal plan		Macronutrient split	C	P	F
Meal 1	200g extra-lean buffalo mince, 40g walnuts, 100g spinach		8	50	30
Meal 2	180g trout, 25g extra virgin olive oil, 100g green beans		4	40	33
Meal 3	180g wild Alaskan salmon, 30g coconut oil, 100g kale		0	44	32
Meal 4	200g lean turkey mince, 50g almond butter, 100g cauliflower		4	60	30
Meal 5	225g cod fillet, 100g basmati rice, 100g string beans		75	44	2
Pre bed	100g oats, 50g whey protein, greens powder		65	50	10
			156	288	137

FAT-LOSS PLANS: WEEK 1

Macro targets: 2,500 kcal, 300g pro/70g fat/160g cho

- The guidelines are based on a ~200lb male at approximately 12–13 per cent body fat, with a caloric maintenance of 3,000 kcal.
- Vegetables were not included in macronutrient intake. Every meal was standardised to 100g green vegetables per meal.
- In some cases numbers were rounded to make things more clear.
- All macros and calorie targets were calculated through MyFitnessPal.
- No supplements except BCAAs, whey protein, greens powders and vitargo (in the final week) were used.
- All foods are readily available in supermarkets and butchers.

Assuming the male maintains his bodyweight at 3,000 kcal, we will use a 500 kcal deficit to trigger fat loss in the body, setting the calories at 2,500 kcal.

For those wanting to adjust to their own bodyweight, the calories and macronutrients were set as follows:

- **Calories:** Maintenance minus 500 kcal, or if unsure of maintenance calories, bodyweight in pounds x 15 as a guideline.
- **Protein:** 1.5g/lb
- **Fats and Carbohydrates:** split 50/50 to make up the remaining calories.

Training days: 4 days a week (e.g. Mon/Tues/Thurs/Fri)

Rationale: Kept protein and fats prior to training. Setting a high protein intake of 1.5g/lb will allow for maximal protection of muscle mass, as well as optimising protein synthesis while in a calorie deficit. Coconut oil is used in pre-training meal for training energy. Carbohydrates primarily utilised post training and the two meals following to maximise the post-workout anabolic window and take advantage of increased GLUT 4 translocation. No post-workout carbohydrate powders are taken, to allow greater satiety and volume of food when dieting.

Rest days: 3 days a week

Rationale: Primarily protein and fats for first three meals in the day to help with increasing insulin sensitivity throughout the day as well as allowing increased fat oxidation. The majority of carbohydrates are in the last three meals of the day. While dieting and on a low carbohydrate intake, this strategy can be beneficial for sleep quality. In addition, carbohydrates at night will top up glycogen stores for the next day's session, especially as very few carbohydrates will be consumed pre workout, as well as ensuring performance is kept high in the gym. The set-up can be adapted so that the first two meals are protein and fats followed by the three carbohydrate meals, before ending with protein and fats. Choosing between the two can be individual to the person. People who find they sleep well off carbohydrates can choose the former option, while those who don't can change around.

Monday

Meal plan		Macronutrient split	P	F	C
Meal 1	200g grass-fed beef fillet steak, 25g almonds, 100g spinach		50	30	5
Meal 2	200g cod fillet, 15g coconut oil, 100g broccoli		35	15	0
During	20g BCAA		20	0	0
Post	50g whey protein		40	2	3
Meal 3 (60–90 mins later)	200g prawns, 100g green beans, 60g basmati rice		40	3	47
Meal 4	200g chicken breast, 50g basmati rice, 10ml extra virgin olive oil, 100g cauliflower		50	10	40
Meal 5	200g chicken breast, 100g green beans, 100g oatmeal		65	10	65
			303	70	160

Tuesday

Meal plan		Macronutrient split	P	F	C
Meal 1	200g venison mince home-made burger, 25g macadamia nuts, 100g spinach		46	26	2
Meal 2	200g line-caught haddock, 15g coconut oil, 100g broccoli		34	15	0
During	20g BCAA		20	0	0
Post	50g whey protein		40	2	3
Meal 3	200g chicken breast, 100g green beans, 250g sweet potato		50	3	50
Meal 4	200g wild-caught tuna, 15g grass-fed butter, 200g sweet potato, 100g broccoli		50	14	40
Meal 5	200g diced turkey breast, 100g mange tout, 100g oatmeal		60	10	65
			300	70	160

Wednesday

Meal plan		Macronutrient split	P	F	C
Meal 1	220g buffalo mince, 15g walnuts, 100g spinach		50	15	5
Meal 2	200g trout, 100g green beans		45	12	5
Meal 3	200g wild Alaskan salmon, ½ medium avocado		50	25	8
Meal 4	250g cod fillet, 60g basmati rice, 100g broccoli		50	2	45
Meal 5	200g turkey mince, 75g quinoa, 100g green beans		55	8	47
Pre bed	75g oatmeal, 50g whey, greens powder		50	8	50
			300	70	160

Thursday

Meal plan		Macronutrient split	P	F	C
Meal 1	200g grass-fed fillet steak, 30g cashew butter, 100g spinach		50	30	5
Meal 2	200g cod fillet, 10g coconut oil, 100g broccoli		35	12	0
During	20g BCAA		20	0	0
Post	50g whey protein		40	2	3
Meal 3	200g chicken breast, 100g green beans, 60g jasmine rice		50	2	50
Meal 4	200g chicken breast, 10ml extra virgin olive oil, 50g jasmine rice, 100g peppers		50	12	40
Meal 5	200g turkey mince, 100g romaine lettuce, 100g oatmeal		55	12	62
			300	70	160

Friday

Meal plan		Macronutrient split	P	F	C
Meal 1	200g grass-fed extra-lean beef mince, 40g Brazil nuts, 100g spinach		50	35	2
Meal 2	200g line-caught plaice, 15g coconut oil, 100g broccoli		45	20	0
During	20g BCAA		20	0	0
Post	50g whey protein		40	2	3
Meal 3	200g prawns, 100g green beans, 250g sweet potato		40	2	55
Meal 4	200g wild-caught tuna, 100g broccoli, 200g sweet potato		50	2	40
Meal 5	200g chicken breast, 100g sugar snap peas, 100g oatmeal		55	9	60
			306	70	160

Saturday

Meal plan		Macronutrient split	P	F	C
Meal 1	2 unsmoked bacon rashers, 4 medium eggs, 100g spinach		34	24	0
Meal 2	200g sardines (tinned), 100g green beans		43	18	0
Meal 3	200g wild-caught salmon, 100g kale		50	9	0
Meal 4	200g chicken breast, 60g basmati rice, 100g broccoli		50	2	45
Meal 5	200g turkey mince, 75g quinoa, 100g green beans		55	7	47
Pre bed	170g 0% fat Greek yoghurt, 50g whey protein, 100g oats		68	10	68
			300	70	160

Sunday

Meal plan		Macronutrient split	P	F	C
Meal 1	200g lamb leg steak, 2 medium eggs, 100g spinach		55	24	0
Meal 2	200g skinless chicken thighs, 100g green beans		37	20	0
Meal 3	200g wild-caught salmon, 100g kale		50	8	0
Meal 4	200g wild-caught tuna, 200g sweet potato, 100g broccoli		50	2	40
Meal 5	150g turkey mince burgers, 85g quinoa, 100g green beans		43	8	52
Pre bed	170g 0% fat Greek yoghurt, 45g whey protein, 100g oats		65	8	68
			300	70	160

FAT-LOSS PLANS: WEEK 2

Macro targets: 2,500 kcal, 300g pro/90g fat/110g cho

This week we will keep protein the same, but will take away 50g of carbohydrates and increase fat to ensure the 2,500 kcal calorie target is reached.

Training days:

With the decrease in carbohydrates, one of the carbohydrate meals is dropped in favour of protein and fat only. Carbohydrates are placed in the post-workout meal and before bed. The latter is to help with sleep during the lower carbohydrate phase and energy deficit.

Rest days:

One of the carbohydrate meals is replaced with a protein and fat only meal, meaning only the last two meals of the day include carbohydrates. While they can be spread throughout the day, the low amount prescribed (110g) would mean having them in two meals only, which would provide more volume of food to eat at each sitting.

Monday

Meal plan	Macronutrient split	P	F	C
Meal 1	200g grass-fed beef fillet steak, 40g almonds, 100g spinach	55	35	7
Meal 2	200g cod fillet, 20g coconut oil, 100g broccoli	35	20	0
During	20g BCAA	20	0	0
Post	50g whey protein	40	2	3
Meal 3	200g prawns, 100g green beans, 60g basmati rice	40	3	45
(60–90 mins later)				
Meal 4	200g chicken breast, 20ml extra virgin olive oil, 100g cauliflower	50	20	0
Meal 5	200g chicken breast, 100g green beans, 80g oatmeal	60	10	55
		300	90	110

Tuesday

Meal plan		Macronutrient split	P	F	C
Meal 1	200g venison mince home-made burger, 40g macadamia nuts, 100g spinach		46	37	4
Meal 2	200g line-caught haddock, 20g coconut oil, 100g broccoli		34	20	0
During	20g BCAA		20	0	0
Post	50g whey protein		40	2	3
Meal 3	200g chicken breast, 100g green beans, 250g sweet potato		50	3	50
Meal 4	200g wild-caught tuna, 20g grass-fed butter, 100g broccoli		50	18	0
Meal 5	200g diced turkey breast, 100g mange tout, 80g oatmeal		60	10	53
			300	90	110

Wednesday

Meal plan		Macronutrient split	P	F	C
Meal 1	230g buffalo mince, 40g walnuts, 100g spinach		56	30	8
Meal 2	200g trout, 100g green beans		45	12	5
Meal 3	200g wild Alaskan salmon, 5g grass-fed butter, 100g mange tout		50	13	0
Meal 4	250g cod fillet, ½ medium avocado, 100g broccoli		47	18	7
Meal 5	200g turkey mince, 65g quinoa, 100g green beans		52	8	40
Pre bed	75g oatmeal, 50g whey protein, greens powder		50	8	50
			300	89	110

Thursday

Meal plan		Macronutrient split	P	F	C
Meal 1	200g grass-fed fillet steak, 40g cashew butter, 100g spinach		51	35	5
Meal 2	200g cod fillet, 20g coconut oil, 100g broccoli		36	21	0
During	20g BCAA		20	0	0
Post	50g whey protein		40	2	3
Meal 3	200g chicken breast, 100g green beans, 65g jasmine rice		50	2	52
Meal 4	200g chicken breast, 20ml extra virgin olive oil, 100g peppers		50	20	0
Meal 5	200g turkey mince, 100g romaine lettuce, 80g oatmeal		53	10	50
			300	90	110

Friday

Meal plan		Macronutrient split	P	F	C
Meal 1	220g grass-fed extra-lean beef mince, 40g Brazil nuts, 100g spinach		50	37	2
Meal 2	200g line-caught plaice, 20g coconut oil, 100g broccoli		45	25	0
During	20g BCAA		20	0	0
Post	50g whey protein		40	2	3
Meal 3	200g prawns, 100g green beans, 250g sweet potato		40	2	55
Meal 4	200g wild-caught tuna, 100g broccoli, 15ml extra virgin olive oil		50	16	0
Meal 5	200g chicken breast, 100g sugar snap peas, 80g oatmeal		55	8	50
			300	90	110

Saturday

Meal plan		Macronutrient split	P	F	C
Meal 1	4 unsmoked bacon rashers, 4 medium eggs, 100g spinach		40	33	0
Meal 2	200g sardines (tinned), 100g green beans		43	18	0
Meal 3	200g wild-caught salmon, 100g kale		50	9	0
Meal 4	200g chicken breast, 10ml extra virgin olive oil, 100g broccoli		45	12	0
Meal 5	200g turkey mince, 65g quinoa, 100g green beans		54	8	42
Pre bed	170g 0% fat Greek yoghurt, 50g whey protein, 100g oats		68	10	68
			300	90	110

Sunday

Meal plan		Macronutrient split	P	F	C
Meal 1	200g lamb leg steak, 2 medium eggs, 100g spinach		55	25	0
Meal 2	200g skinless chicken thighs, 100g green beans		37	20	0
Meal 3	200g wild-caught salmon, 100g kale		50	8	0
Meal 4	200g wild-caught tuna, ½ medium avocado, 100g broccoli		50	21	8
Meal 5	150g turkey mince burgers, 60g quinoa, 100g green beans		41	6	38
Pre bed	170g 0% fat Greek yoghurt, 50g whey protein, 90g oats		67	10	64
			300	90	110

FAT-LOSS PLANS: WEEK 3

Macro targets: 2,500 kcal, 200g pro/55g fat/300g cho

Week 3 brings a large shift in the macronutrient ratios, with a high-carbohydrate, moderate-protein and low-fat approach taken, factored into the same calorie deficit as weeks 1 and 2.

Protein: 1g/lb | Carbohydrates: 1.5g/lb | Fat: Remaining calories within the calorie goal

Training days:
Generally, the same philosophy in terms of nutrient timing is utilised in this week, but with higher volumes of carbohydrate foods, and reduced protein and fat sources. The only notable difference in timing is the addition of berries to breakfast to help achieve the daily carbohydrate goal.

Rest days: 3 days a week
Breakfast remains low-carb to help with managing insulin sensitivity and heighten your body's use of fat as fuel during the day. However, this week all the remaining meals in the day are mixed meals, with the carbohydrates spread evenly through the day, finishing with a slightly higher serving before bed. A strong focus on using low-density carbohydrates (e.g. sweet potato) on rest days will provide more volume of food during a calorie deficit, as well as to help keep blood sugar levels constant.

Monday

Meal plan		Macronutrient split	P	F	C
Meal 1	150g grass-fed beef fillet steak, 20g almonds, 100g blueberries, 100g spinach		40	23	18
Meal 2	150g cod fillet, 15g coconut oil, 100g broccoli		27	15	0
During	10g BCAA		10	0	0
Post	35g whey protein		28	2	2
Meal 3 (60–90 mins later)	150g prawns, 120g jasmine rice, 100g green beans		37	2	90
Meal 4	100g chicken breast, 120g basmati rice, 100g cauliflower		33	2	90
Meal 5	150g oats		25	11	100
			200	55	300

Tuesday

Meal plan		Macronutrient split	P	F	C
Meal 1	150g venison mince home-made burger, 25g macadamia nuts, 100g strawberries, 100g spinach		36	24	18
Meal 2	150g line-caught haddock, 15g coconut oil, 100g broccoli		26	15	0
During	10g BCAA		10	0	0
Post	35g whey protein		28	2	2
Meal 3	120g chicken breast, 120g jasmine rice, 100g green beans		38	1	90
Meal 4	100g tuna steak, 120g basmati rice, 100g broccoli		37	2	90
Meal 5	150g oats		25	11	100
			200	55	300

Wednesday

Meal plan		Macronutrient split	P	F	C
Meal 1	175g buffalo mince, ½ medium avocado, 100g spinach		38	20	10
Meal 2	120g chicken breast, 80g quinoa, 100g green beans		38	5	50
Meal 3	150g wild Alaskan salmon, 250g sweet potato, 100g mange tout		41	6	50
Meal 4	150g cod fillet, 80g quinoa, 100g broccoli		37	5	50
Meal 5	100g turkey mince, 250g sweet potato, 10g butter, 100g green beans		26	10	50
Pre bed	120g oats, 20g sultanas		20	9	80
			200	55	290

Thursday

Meal plan		Macronutrient split	P	F	C
Meal 1	200g grass-fed fillet steak, 20g cashew butter, 100g blueberries, 100g spinach		45	24	18
Meal 2	130g cod fillet, 15g coconut oil, 100g broccoli		23	15	0
During	10g BCAA		10	0	0
Post	35g whey protein		28	2	2
Meal 3	120g chicken breast, 120g jasmine rice, 100g green beans		37	1	90
Meal 4	100g chicken breast, 120g basmati rice, 100g peppers		32	2	90
Meal 5	150g oatmeal		25	11	100
			200	55	300

Friday

Meal plan		Macronutrient split	P	F	C
Meal 1	220g grass-fed extra-lean beef mince, 40g Brazil nuts, 100g spinach		40	22	18
Meal 2	150g line-caught plaice, 15g coconut oil, 100g broccoli		27	17	0
During	10g BCAA		10	0	0
Post	35g whey protein		28	2	2
Meal 3	150g prawns, 120g jasmine rice, 100g green beans		33	2	90
Meal 4	120g wild-caught tuna, 120g basmati rice, 100g broccoli		37	1	90
Meal 5	150g oatmeal		25	11	100
			200	55	300

Saturday

Meal plan		Macronutrient split	P	F	C
Meal 1	2 unsmoked bacon rashers, 4 medium eggs, 100g spinach		34	24	0
Meal 2	120g chicken breast, 80g quinoa, 100g green beans		38	5	50
Meal 3	150g wild-caught salmon, 250g sweet potato, 100g kale		41	6	50
Meal 4	120g chicken breast, 80g quinoa, 100g broccoli		38	6	50
Meal 5	100g turkey mince, 250g sweet potato, 5g grass-fed butter, 100g green beans		26	5	50
Pre bed	130g oatmeal, 20g sultanas		23	9	100
			200	55	300

Sunday

Meal plan		Macronutrient split	P	F	C
Meal 1	150g lamb leg steak, 2 medium eggs, 100g spinach		45	22	0
Meal 2	100g turkey mince burgers, 80g quinoa 100g green beans		30	7	50
Meal 3	150g wild-caught salmon, 250g sweet potato, 100g kale		40	6	50
Meal 4	120g wild-caught tuna, 80g quinoa, 100g broccoli		36	6	50
Meal 5	100g turkey mince burgers, 250g sweet potato, 5g grass-fed butter, 100g green beans		26	5	50
Pre bed	130g oatmeal, 20g sultanas		23	9	100
			200	55	300

FAT-LOSS PLANS: WEEK 4

This week we will keep the same 2,500 kcal deficit, but introduce some aggressive carb cycling into the plan in order to ramp up your fat-loss efforts.

Macro targets:
Monday: 300g pro/120g fat/50g cho
Tuesday: 300g pro/120g fat/50g cho
Wednesday: 250g pro/55g fat/250g cho
Thursday: 300g pro/75g fat/150g cho
Friday: 300g pro/120g fat/50g cho
Saturday: 300g pro/110g fat/75g cho
Sunday: 150g pro/35g fat/400g cho

Monday

Meal plan		Macronutrient split	P	F	C
Meal 1	200g grass-fed beef fillet steak, 40g almonds, 100g spinach		55	35	7
Meal 2	200g cod fillet, 20g coconut oil, 100g broccoli		35	20	0
During	20g BCAA		20	0	0
Post	40g whey protein		32	2	2
Meal 3	200g prawns, 100g green beans, 200g sweet potato		40	3	38
(60–90 mins later)					
Meal 4	150g chicken breast, 3 medium eggs. 15ml extra virgin olive oil, 100g cauliflower		58	30	0
Meal 5	200g chicken breast, 50g almond butter, 100g green beans		60	30	3
			300	120	50

Tuesday

Meal plan		Macronutrient split	P	F	C
Meal 1	200g venison mince home-made burger, 50g macadamia nuts, 100g spinach		48	45	5
Meal 2	200g line-caught haddock, 20g coconut oil, 100g broccoli		35	20	0
During	20g BCAA		20	0	0
Post	40g whey protein		32	2	2
Meal 3	200g wild-caught tuna, 100g green beans, 200g sweet potato		53	2	40
Meal 4	200g chicken breast, 3 medium eggs, 15ml extra virgin olive oil, 100g broccoli		58	28	0
Meal 5	200g turkey diced breast, 30g peanut butter, 100g mange tout		53	23	3
			299	120	50

Wednesday

Meal plan		Macronutrient split	P	F	C
Meal 1	200g buffalo mince, ½ medium avocado, 100g spinach		44	20	10
Meal 2	175g chicken breast, 70g quinoa, 100g green beans		49	6	45
Meal 3	150g wild Alaskan salmon, 250g sweet potato, 100g mange tout		41	6	50
Meal 4	175g cod fillet, 70g quinoa, 100g broccoli		41	6	45
Meal 5	150g turkey mince, 250g sweet potato, 10g grass-fed butter, 100g green beans		37	11	50
Pre bed	35g whey protein, 60g oats, 10g sultanas		38	6	50
			250	55	250

Thursday

Meal plan		Macronutrient split	P	F	C
Meal 1	200g grass-fed fillet steak, 20g cashew butter, 100g blueberries, 100g spinach		52	29	18
Meal 2	200g cod fillet, 15g coconut oil, 100g broccoli		36	15	0
During	20g BCAA		20	0	0
Post	40g whey protein		32	2	2
Meal 3	200g chicken breast, 100g green beans, 80g jasmine rice		52	2	64
Meal 4	200g chicken breast, 15ml extra virgin olive oil, 100g peppers		46	16	0
Meal 5	200g turkey mince, 100g romaine lettuce, 100g oatmeal		62	11	66
			300	75	150

Friday

Meal plan		Macronutrient split	P	F	C
Meal 1	220g grass-fed extra-lean beef mince, 50g Brazil nuts, 100g spinach		50	45	2
Meal 2	250g line-caught plaice, 20g coconut oil, 100g broccoli		45	25	0
During	20g BCAA		20	0	0
Post	50g whey protein		40	2	3
Meal 3	200g prawns, 100g green beans, 220g sweet potato		40	2	43
Meal 4	200g wild-caught tuna, 3 medium eggs, 10ml extra virgin olive oil, 100g broccoli		50	23	0
Meal 5	200g chicken breast, 30g hazelnut butter, 100g sugar snap peas		55	22	2
			300	119	50

Saturday

Meal plan		Macronutrient split	P	F	C
Meal 1	4 unsmoked bacon rashers, 4 medium eggs, 100g spinach		40	33	0
Meal 2	200g lamb leg steaks, 10g coconut oil, 100g green beans		40	26	0
Meal 3	200g wild-caught salmon, 20g walnuts, 100g kale		52	22	1
Meal 4	200g chicken breast, ½ medium avocado, 100g broccoli		50	18	8
Meal 5	200g turkey mince, 10g grass-fed butter, 100g green beans		46	12	0
Pre bed	170g 0% fat Greek yoghurt, 50g whey protein, 85g oats		72	9	66
			300	120	75

Sunday

Meal plan		Macronutrient split	P	F	C
Meal 1	100g beef fillet steak, 10g coconut oil, 100g blueberries, 100g spinach		29	13	14
Meal 2	100g lean turkey mince, 100g gluten-free penne pasta, 100g green beans		28	4	77
Meal 3	100g wild-caught tuna, 5g grass-fed butter, 100g basmati rice		33	6	77
Meal 4	70g oatmeal, 20g sultanas		13	5	60
Meal 5	100g lean turkey mince, 100g gluten-free penne pasta, 100g green beans		28	4	77
Pre bed	Rice pudding: 75g basmati rice, 300ml skimmed milk, 1 small banana		19	1	95
			150	33	400

FAT-LOSS PLANS: WEEK 5 PEAK WEEK

So, the peak week! When the hard work is done and you have followed the above protocols to achieve the low levels of body fat you desire, whether it has been for 4 or 16 weeks, there are a few things you can do at the end to maximise the look of your physique. Remember, before following this, you must be lean and in a state of 'depletion' to actually warrant this week, otherwise there will be little benefit to it.

Please bear in mind this is a generic plan, and one that can be adapted depending on how lean you are, how you deal with specific macronutrient ratios, and a whole host of other factors. The following is to give you an idea of how you may lay out a 'peak week'.

There will be no water or sodium manipulations, as these should be kept at normal levels throughout the week. On the day there are some slight adjustments, which can be seen below.

It is important to note that the template is very flexible, and should not be written in stone, if you're lean enough, as everyone will react differently and may need more or less food.

The training days have been adjusted to Mon/Wed/Thurs/Fri, with the latter three days being lighter 'pump' days to allow for more efficient calorie (in particular carbohydrate) assimilation and nutrient uptake on the loading days.

Macro targets:
Monday: 275g pro/70g fat/150g cho
Tuesday: 275g pro/70g fat/150g cho
Wednesday: 225g pro/90g fat/450g cho
Thursday: 225g pro/90g fat/300g cho
Friday: 225g pro/90g fat/200g cho
Saturday: 225g pro/90g fat/200g cho
Sunday: no macros, sample day plan below

Monday

Meal plan		Macronutrient split	P	F	C
Meal 1	200g grass-fed beef fillet steak, 25g almonds, 100g spinach		50	30	5
Meal 2	200g cod fillet, 15g coconut oil, 100g broccoli		35	16	0
During	20g BCAA		20	0	0
Post	40g whey protein		32	2	2
Meal 3 (60–90 mins later)	200g prawns, 100g green beans, 60g basmati rice		40	3	47
Meal 4	175g chicken breast, 10ml extra virgin olive oil, 60g basmati rice, 100g cauliflower		45	12	46
Meal 5	175g chicken breast, 100g green beans, 100g oatmeal		53	7	50
			275	70	150

Tuesday

Meal plan		Macronutrient split	P	F	C
Meal 1	200g buffalo mince, 15g walnuts, 100g spinach		44	15	5
Meal 2	200g trout, 100g green beans		42	10	0
Meal 3	200g wild Alaskan salmon, ½ medium avocado		40	22	8
Meal 4	250g cod fillet, 60g basmati rice, 100g broccoli		41	3	46
Meal 5	200g turkey mince, 75g quinoa, 100g green beans		54	12	42
Pre bed	75g oatmeal, 50g whey, greens powder		52	8	49
			273	70	150

Wednesday

Meal plan		Macronutrient split	P	F	C
Meal 1	175g beef fillet steak, 15g coconut oil, 100g blueberries, 100g spinach		50	22	14
During training	20g BCAA, 40g Vitargo		20	0	40
Meal 2 (60–90 mins later)	150g lean turkey mince, 100g gluten-free penne pasta, 100g green beans		39	5	76
Meal 3	150g wild-caught tuna, 20ml extra virgin olive oil, 100g basmati rice		45	20	76
Meal 4	70g oatmeal, 20g sultanas, 40g 85% dark chocolate		17	26	73
Meal 5	150g lamb leg steak, 100g gluten-free penne pasta, 100g green beans		35	16	76
Pre bed	Rice pudding: 75g basmati rice, 300ml skimmed milk, 1 small banana		19	1	95
			225	90	450

Thursday

Meal plan		Macronutrient split (P	F	C)
Meal 1	150g grass-fed fillet steak, 40g cashew butter, 100g blueberries, 100g spinach	44	31	20
Meal 2	150g cod fillet, 15g coconut oil, 100g broccoli	27	15	0
During training	20g BCAA, 40g Vitargo	20	0	40
Meal 3	150g chicken breast, 100g jasmine rice, 100g green beans	42	2	80
Meal 4	150g chicken breast, 100g basmati rice, 20ml extra virgin olive oil, 100g peppers	44	21	77
Meal 5	100g oatmeal, 35g whey protein, 20g 85% dark chocolate, 15g sultanas	48	21	83
		225	90	300

Friday

Meal plan		Macronutrient split P	F	C
Meal 1	200g grass-fed extra-lean beef mince, 40g Brazil nuts, 100g spinach	48	36	1
Meal 2	250g line-caught plaice, 15g coconut oil, 100g broccoli	45	19	0
During training	20g BCAA, 20g Vitargo	20	0	20
Meal 3	200g prawns, 250g sweet potato, 100g green beans	33	2	50
Meal 4	120g wild-caught tuna, 3 medium eggs, 250g sweet potato, 100g broccoli	56	13	50
Meal 5	120g oatmeal, 20g hazelnut butter	23	20	80
		225	90	201

Saturday

Meal plan		Macronutrient split P	F	C
Meal 1	150g beef fillet steak, 10g coconut oil, 100g spinach	35	22	0
Meal 2	100g turkey mince burgers, 25g almond butter, 100g green beans	33	16	2
Meal 3	150g wild-caught salmon, 250g sweet potato, 100g kale	41	6	50
Meal 4	120g wild-caught tuna, 60g basmati rice	41	16	47
Meal 5	120g chicken breast, 60g basmati rice, 10ml extra virgin olive oil	33	11	47
Pre bed	150g lamb leg steak, 80g oats	42	19	54
		225	90	200

PEAK DAY

Now that you've reached the day you've been peaking for, there are a few little tricks we can use on the day to maximise your physique's fullness and muscularity. There are no specific macros, as it is done very much by feel and how you look at the time (as the week should be, in particular the latter part).

Choose foods you digest well, as risking any foods you may be intolerant to at this point can trigger bloating. As you may have realised, vegetables were dropped halfway through the day before (Saturday), and low-fibre foods were chosen. This is to reduce any possibility of gut filling, which may help with improved abdominal presentation.

Lastly, a good choice on this day is to have a high-carb/fat/sodium mix approx two to three hours before you want to 'peak' for your photos/event, as this can help fill out your muscles, and help with pumping up.

Sample plan

Meal 1 (8 hours before)	100–150g red meat, 1 small banana, 60g oats, 500ml water
Meal 2 (6 hours before)	100g chicken, 60g rice, 500ml water
Meal 3 (4 hours before)	100g chicken, 60g rice. From now, sips of water to quench thirst
Meal 4 (2 hours before)	Protein/carb/fat/sodium meal mix. A pizza or a sub are great options
30 mins before	2 rice cakes with hazelnut and chocolate spread/peanut butter and jelly (fast-acting sugars and fat)
Just before/during	Small chocolate bar/jelly sweets (fast-acting sugars)

08

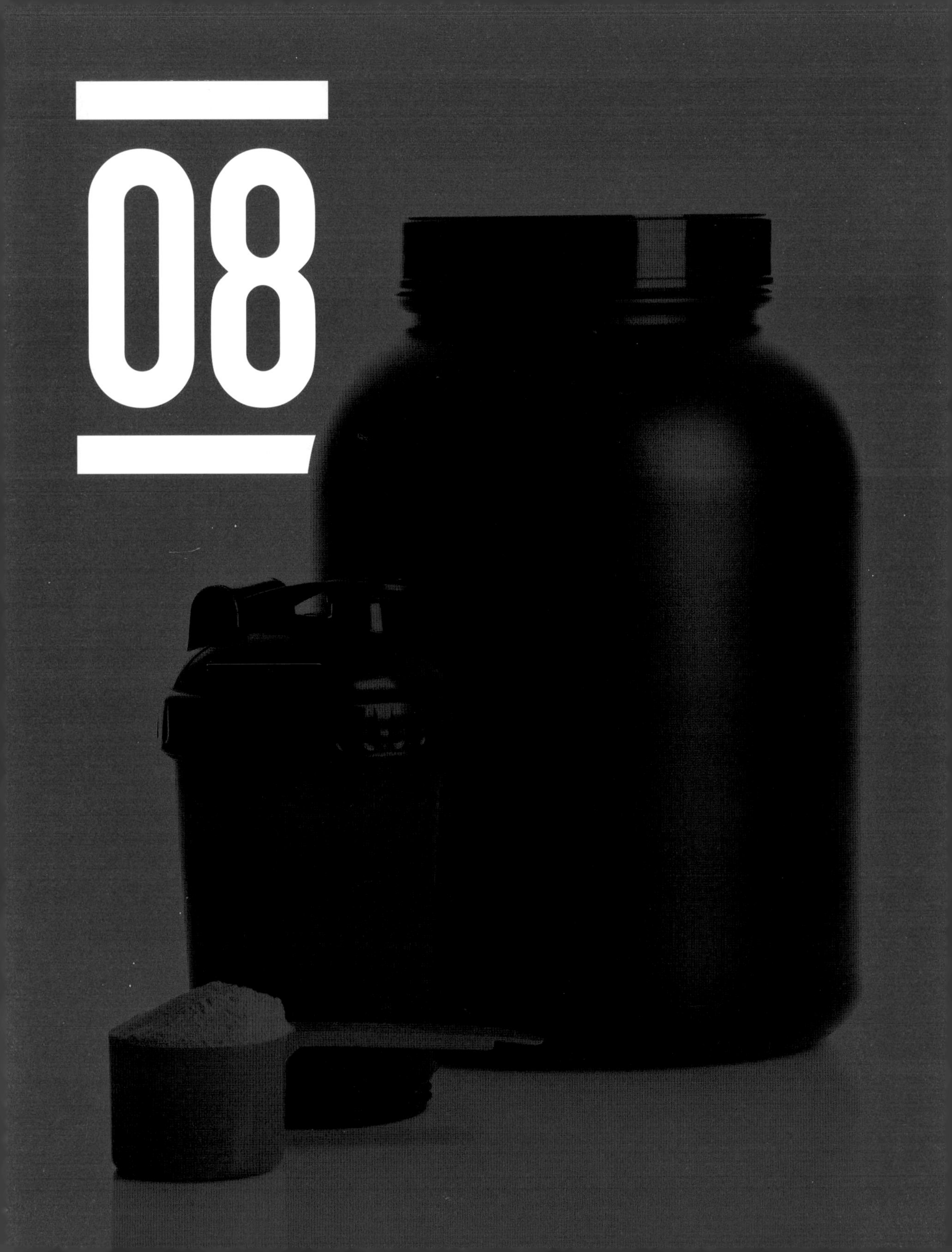

SUPPLEMENTS
AND
NUTRACEUTICALS

Your route to better results or expensive urine? I've never encountered a trainee who obsesses over supplements more than his diet who is happy with his results. Food, exercise and lifestyle are the foundation; supplements are just the window-dressing after the house has been built.

There are two reasons why too many of us are obsessed with the use of nutritional supplements. Get your head around the reasons why this is the case and you will have taken the first step to a controlled, measured and appropriate use of these often controversial products.

1. SUPPLEMENTS ARE BIG BUSINESS

If I wanted to make the most amount of money in the shortest possible time I would quit the gym/personal training business and put all my efforts into creating a supplement brand.

The margins are eye-wateringly good, the barriers to entry minuscule and there is (sadly) a sucker born every minute.

Did you know that almost all of the protein powder sold by UK sports nutrition companies comes from the same Irish manufacturers? Far too often we are paying a premium for a fancy label and some extravagant marketing claims.

The fitness magazines are propped up by supplement company advertising revenue so the unsuspecting public gets relentlessly bombarded with endless messages about the vital importance of supplements.

This is BS.

Supplements can be a hugely useful tool and my own supplement cupboard is always well stocked. But they are a tertiary consideration that falls behind every other factor featured in this book.

If truth be told I did not even want to put this chapter in because there is always the risk that you, dear reader, will place too great an emphasis on supplements and waste your time and money by getting your priorities wrong.

2. EVERYONE WANTS A SHORTCUT

Supplements, especially with the invasive and clever marketing perpetuated by their manufacturers, speak to the lazy and impatient person who lurks inside all of us.

Everyone wants to follow the line of least resistance and get to their goal as swiftly and painlessly as possible. The latest 'better than steroids' pill, powder or potion often feels like something that we miss out on at our peril.

I've made all the mistakes and fallen hook, line and sinker for so much grandiose hyperbole that I dread to think of the money wasted.

I don't want you to make the same mistakes that I have made.

NOW THAT YOU ARE THOROUGHLY DEPRESSED

If you are now looking at your own protein powder stash and feeling despondent, snap out of it.

All of the above qualifications aside, there are still many great supplement products out there – just do not forget that they are designed to supplement, not replace, a balanced, varied and healthy diet comprising real, whole food.

No supplement is a shortcut to success.

You need to train, eat and rest as well as possible because that is the key to a successful transformation. If you are doing these three things right, then supplements may have a role to play in accelerating your journey to the finish.

Just be aware that the scientific research on some of these supplements is a bit hazy, to say the least. That's because controlled, large-scale human studies are expensive, and extremely difficult to control properly.

That said, the following supplements are included in this book because I believe – through my own anecdotal experience, as a trainee, a trainer and the owner of UP observing the results of thousands of results-oriented personal training clients – that they are of benefit to you in getting to where you want to be.

That's no guarantee that one or any of them will work for you. There is no silver bullet for instant success. But in my experience they can make a difference, so long as you are training, eating and resting well.

SUPPLEMENT BRAND QUALITY

Supplement quality is a minefield, and knowing which company to trust versus which company uses fillers, weak and watered-down 'proprietary formulas', or just tells outright lies, is incredibly tough for the layman.

I could give you a list of my own most trusted supplement companies but the danger in doing that is that by the time you read this that company may have changed beyond all recognition. If you think I am being dramatic look no further than how the Gaspari brand fell from on high after lab results showed that their protein powder contained half the protein that the label claimed!

And then we have the all-too-common practice with many companies of 'amino spiking' in their protein powders. While this sounds like quite a cool new benefit for your protein it actually means that certain unscrupulous manufacturers were spiking their powders with cheap amino acids, such as glycine and taurine, in order to give a higher overall protein reading.

If you want to know the supplement companies who I feel represent the best and most up to date in quality and value then drop me a line on Twitter (@HeyNickMitchell) or go to www.UltimateTransformation.Guide where I will keep a time-stamped list of my current recommendations.

PINPOINTING THE SUPPLEMENTS YOU NEED

Taking supplements that you don't need is unlikely to harm you, but it is going to lighten your wallet and leave you with expensive urine.

In an ideal world I'd do what we do with UP's personal training clients and send you to a laboratory to run a series of blood tests. However, I realise that this isn't practical or within the budget of most readers. So how do you decide what you should be taking?

The best solution is to try one product at a time and monitor how you respond. If your digestion is better, or your sleep is improved, then for me that's a tick in the box and the product should be kept in your supplement arsenal. However, I have never met a single man who is hell-bent on transforming his physique with the patience to adopt that approach. I know for certain that there's no chance I could do it myself!

To help you decide if a supplement is right for you I've given it a score. Does this mean that the highest-scoring supplements are right for you? No – you'll have to read the text to decide if experimenting with it fits your goals. And a low score in one category doesn't mean the product is 'bad', just not as useful. For example, a lower health score does not mean a supplement is unhealthy – far from it – but it does mean that it has fewer direct health benefits.

And if I can give you one parting thought it is this: supplements have never created a single body transformation, but good food has been the key to every result I've ever worked with. Please allow that fact to sink in before getting out your credit card.

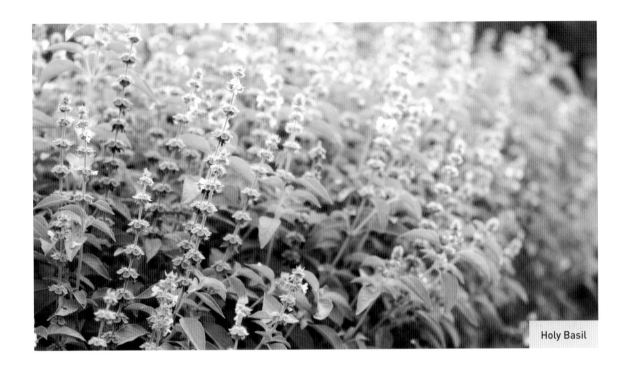

Holy Basil

THE TOP SUPPLEMENTS AND NUTRACEUTICALS

BCAAs

WHAT? BCAAs, or branched-chain amino acids to give them their proper name, are taken during heavy weight training. Each capsule contains the ideal anabolic (muscle-building) ratio of the three amino acids leucine, isoleucine and valine.
WHEN? During your workout.
WHY? Taking these during your workout has numerous benefits, including preventing muscle tissue breakdown and post-workout soreness and increasing post-workout muscle recovery and testosterone levels.

Health: 2/20
Performance: 19/20
Body composition: 15/20
OVERALL: 36/60

BETA-ALANINE

WHAT? A type of beta amino acid.
WHEN? About 30 minutes before training.
Stick to label guidelines for dosage.
WHY? This supplement is great for improving focus and concentration during your session. It increases carnosine concentration in the

muscle, allowing for improved performance by buffering hydrogen ions during intense exercise, such as weight training, but not cardio.

Health: 1/20
Performance: 17/20
Body composition: 10/20
OVERALL: 28/60

CREATINE

WHAT?The back-up generator for your muscles.
WHEN? Take 5g in your post-workout shake to replenish lost stores or split your dose and have half prior to your workout and half after. And drink plenty of water: creatine is hygroscopic, so it'll suck water into your muscles and can leave you dehydrated.
WHY? Our body metabolises creatine into ATP, which is used for every initial muscle movement. It's therefore vital to have adequate supplies during heavy, high-intensity workouts to deliver the required energy to your muscles. In other words, creatine helps you lift harder for longer.

Put simply, creatine works. It is cheap, it has been proven to be good for your muscles

and your brain, and it helps you lift more weight, which allows you to lay down more new muscle tissue. There's a lot of controversy regarding creatine esters and loading, and my two cents is to just keep it very simple. Stick with the basic creatine monohydrate variation and use 5g (a teaspoonful) in a post-workout shake. On non-training days add it to a drink in the morning so that it is easier to remember to take it.

Health: 15/20
Performance: 15/20
Body composition: 15/20
OVERALL: 45/60

D3

WHAT? Think of D3 not as a vitamin but as an immune system regulating hormone.
WHEN? 10,000–25,000 IU twice a week.
WHY? The harsh fact is that almost all of us are deficient in this absolutely vital substance and, as you may have gathered by now, most of what we want from any supplement intake is to optimise health even if body composition is the only

goal (which sounds kind of an odd goal to me as they should go hand-in-hand if you are a sane and rational person). Optimal health leads to a better-functioning body that is much more capable of putting in stellar gym performances and losing body fat and gaining muscle. Many studies also suggest that vitamin D may decrease risk for many diseases and conditions including certain types of cancer, multiple sclerosis, hypertension, weight loss and even longevity.

D3 is actually fairly simple to test for and most doctors will do it for you if you ask them nicely. The test is called a 25 Hydroxy-Vitamin D Test and most forward-thinking health experts seem to be recommending an optimal level of between 60 and 80ng/ml. If you are in the UK then converting the numbers your doctor is most likely to use (nmol/litre) is simply a matter of dividing by 2.5.

Health: 20/20
Performance: 1/20
Body composition: 10/20
OVERALL: 31/60

DIGESTIVE ENZYMES

WHAT? This compound helps your body break down the food you eat more efficiently and effectively.

WHEN? With food.

WHY? Contrary to the popular expression, you are not what you eat. You are in fact what you absorb.

One of my (pet) theories why skinny guys stay skinny is that they do not have the best digestive systems for absorbing all that they need from their food. Digestive enzymes will help alleviate this problem and allow you to utilise your food much more effectively.

Choose a supplement that contains compounds that help you extract vitamin B12 and iron from food, both of which are vital for good energy levels, as well as pepsin, herbal bitter and gentian root, all of which fire up your digestive system.

Health: 15/20
Performance: 1/20
Body composition: 12/20
OVERALL: 28/60

ELECTROLYTES

WHAT? Electrolytes are salts that the body loses through sweating.

WHEN? During exercise, especially higher-intensity sweaty exercise.

WHY? Forget all the fancy pre- and peri-workout drinks. Every one of you who trains hard should consume some extra electrolytes during exercise, and while there are some grand and expensive concoctions out there, cheap electrolyte sachets and/ or rehydration kits abound and more than do the job. When you first use them you may well be very pleasantly surprised at your improved workout stamina.

Just try to avoid the sugar- and/or caffeine-filled sports drinks that are too often pushed out on the unwary consumer. They will be very unlikely to help you do anything other than lighten your wallet.

Health: 14/20
Performance: 20/20
Body composition: 10/20
OVERALL: 44/60

GLUTAMINE

WHAT? The gut-calmer.

WHEN? Taking 10g in water on an empty stomach pre-breakfast will aid in gut healing and function, while 10g post-workout will aid in glutamine store replenishment. Take 30g post-workout if you're on a low-carb diet to enhance glycogen replenishment.

WHY? This amino acid should already be present in your body, but if you have gut issues or you train hard then glutamine could be great for you because it strengthens the lining of your gut and helps protein synthesis.

Health: 18/20
Performance: 5/20
Body composition: 12/20
OVERALL: 35/60

GLUTATHIONE

WHAT? A powerful antioxidant to protect the brain and body tissues from the damage by free radicals. It also acts to recycle vitamins C and E, which also reduce free radicals.

WHEN? Before bed as it is synergistic with melatonin; however, there is one massive caveat here: ingesting glutathione orally will get you nowhere as it is destroyed in the stomach. The best form of delivery is 100–250mg via an intramuscular injection.

WHY? Your body will work much better with higher levels of glutathione. It is used for everything from the treatment of cataracts, cancer, asthma, Parkinson's through to diabetes and assisting in recovery from chemotherapy. It is not a drug, and it should be perceived as one of the most powerful immune system boosters known to man.

Health: 20/20
Performance: 10/20
Body composition: 8/20
OVERALL: 38/60

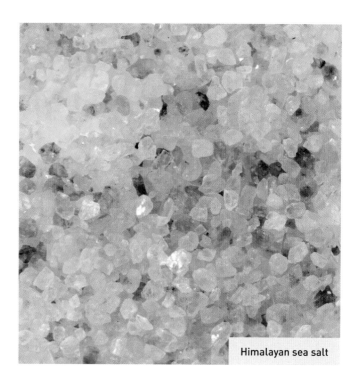
Himalayan sea salt

HIMALAYAN SEA SALT

WHAT? Unprocessed coloured (pink) salt.

WHEN? With food or even ¼ teaspoon in a glass of water first thing in the morning.

WHY? This addition may have surprised you! It isn't really a supplement per se, but you can and should 'supplement' your diet with it. Commercial refined table salt is stripped of most of its minerals, aside from sodium chloride, chemically bleached and laden with additives to prevent it caking.

Himalayan salt can help to create a healthy electrolyte balance, improve hydration, balance pH, improve metabolism, lower blood pressure, and there is even a school of thought that it can help to reset the adrenals.

Health: 10/20
Performance: 1/20
Body composition: 5/20
OVERALL: 16/60

HOLY BASIL

WHAT? An aromatic plant grown in the tropics.

WHEN? Two tablets each with breakfast and lunch.

WHY? Compounds found in holy basil limit your cortisol response when you're faced with those daily disturbances that can make your blood boil. Having high levels of this stress hormone rampaging through your system is very damaging and can result in your body storing more fat around your belly. This supplement will also protect the body from the effects of both physical and chemical stress and will boost morning and afternoon energy.

When building muscle one vital factor to always keep at the forefront of your mind is enhancing the cortisol–testosterone axis in favour of testosterone, the hormone that will do all sorts of amazing things for helping you lay down new muscle tissue. Holy basil is an adaptogenic herb that lifts you up if you are down, and calms you down if you are too 'up', allowing you to better deal with stress and have a more optimally functioning endocrine system. This is probably my personal favourite herbal supplement.

Health: 10/20
Performance: 10/20
Body composition: 10/20
OVERALL: 30/60

L-CARNITINE

WHAT? A compound primarily found in red meat.

WHEN? 500–3,000mg per day, ideally on an empty stomach.

WHY? It plays many roles in the body, specifically in helping to use fat stores as fuel.

Health: 10/20
Performance: 10/20
Body composition: 10/20
OVERALL: 30/60

LOW-OSMOLALITY CARBOHYDRATE POWDERS

WHAT? Low-osmolality/high molecular weight (HMW) carbohydrate powders are carbs that pass rapidly through the stomach with a speed and efficiency that is far superior to regular carb powder products such as dextrose and maltodextrin. The most well-known examples of HMW carbs are branched cyclic dextrin and vitargo.

WHEN? During and/or immediately after your workout, assuming that you are doing enough volume in your training to justify their use and your insulin sensitivity is high enough. A broad rule of thumb is if you can't at least see your top layers of abdominal muscles then you're too fat for intra-workout carbs.

WHY? The osmolality of HMW carbohydrates can potentially speed up the rate of glycogen synthesis post-workout, allowing for decreased catabolism and increased protein synthesis.

The latest kid on the HMW carbs block is 'highly branched cyclic dextrin' (HBCD). It has an even lower osmolality than vitargo and has been used with great success in intra-workout drinks.

Health: 0/20
Performance: 18/20
Body composition: 18/20
OVERALL: 36/60

MAGNESIUM

WHAT? Magnesium is a commonly deficient mineral that is vital for your optimal health and progress.

WHEN? Use before bed as it can aid restful sleep and calm down the nervous system.

WHY? Magnesium is the fourth most abundant mineral in the body and involved in 300 essential biochemical reactions in the body, ranging from energy production in your cells to protein synthesis, making it vital for optimal athletic performance. The majority of adults in the Western world are deficient in magnesium so while it isn't going to make you 'swole', there is a significant chance that you need it.

Health: 20/20
Performance: 5/20
Body composition: 12/20
OVERALL: 37/60

OMEGA-3

WHAT? A type of essential fatty acid.

WHEN? 5g a day.

WHY? Omega-3 is mainly found in oily, cold-water fish, and is essential for good health – research has shown that it

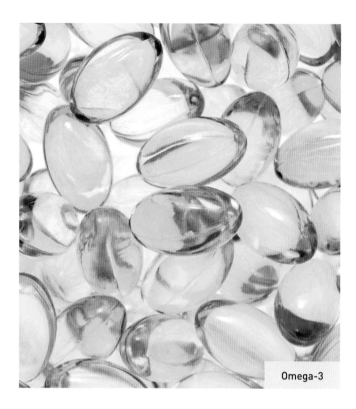

Omega-3

helps prevent a host of serious long-term ailments including cancer and heart disease. It's especially beneficial when trying to lose weight because it promotes the utilisation of existing fat stores for fuel.

If you are really nailing your diet and eating a mix of oily fish and wild meat every day then you can skip supplementing with Omega-3 as you'll already be getting enough in your diet.

Health: 20/20
Performance: 5/20
Body composition: 14/20
OVERALL: 39/60

MULTIVITAMINS

WHAT: The back-up plan.

WHEN? Try to have some consistency when taking this supplement. It makes sense to take them before mealtimes with a glass of water, to aid absorption of their micronutrients.

WHY: Though you shouldn't rely on them to make up for a bad diet, a quality multivitamin can help to fill in the gaps in an otherwise solid eating plan. Deficiencies in vitamins can cause mood swings, depression, lethargy and exhaustion, but taking a daily dose will keep you on the up and focused on your goals.

Health: 16/20
Performance: 5/20
Body composition: 5/20
OVERALL: 26/60

PHOSPHATIDYLSERINE (PS)

WHAT? A phospholipid that helps brain function and can be of huge benefit to the typical, over-thinking, over-worrying, stressed-out hard-gainer.
WHEN? Post-workout to help lower cortisol levels, or my preferred way in a dosage of 400–800mg at night before bed.
WHY? Lowering cortisol levels at the right times (later in the day or after training) is crucial in this over-stressed and over-ramped-up world that we live in. Maximising sleep and balancing out your hormonal system should be a priority for anyone wanting to improve their physique, and PS is a useful tool in helping you achieve this goal.

In the dosage I have recommended, higher than most studies have used, you get a calming effect, possibly from the lowered cortisol, and sleep and rest are improved. For best use, and to keep the cost down if you are on a budget as it isn't the cheapest product in the world, I would use it three nights a week or at times of higher physical or emotional stress.

Health: 4/20
Performance: 8/20
Body composition: 10/20
OVERALL: 22/60

PROBIOTICS

WHAT? Healthy bacteria for your gut.
WHEN? Standard dose is to take 1–2 caps on an empty stomach before breakfast.
WHY? I don't like the typical body-building supplements that all seem to be aimed at making you 'swole' or 'ripped' as their defining purpose. The best way to use most supplements is to optimise your health so that then you have the very best platform from which to build your body. Probiotics are a perfect example of this and in my opinion should be in every single person's supplement cupboard, regardless of goal or fitness/health levels.

Probiotics improve the health of your gut (where up to 80 per cent of your immune health derives from), and these microbiota contribute to crucial factors such as the regulation of fat storage, and numerous other metabolic functions such as the all-important (for muscle building) protein synthesis.

The healthier your gut the easier it is for you to eliminate waste products, such as lactic acid and inflammatory markers caused by training. In turn, you will recover more rapidly and the increased protein synthesis will boost your overall anabolic response.

Health: 20/20
Performance: 1/20
Body composition: 5/20
OVERALL: 26/60

SULBUTIAMINE

WHAT? A synthetic derivative of thiamine (vitamin B1).

WHEN? 20–200mg pre-workout or early in the morning.

WHY? Sulbutiamine is a neurotransmitter potentiator so it reportedly improves many functions in the brain and body. Certainly you should feel more focus and drive when using it, but it has been used in the treatment of chronic fatigue and erectile dysfunction and for improved memory.

Health: 10/20
Performance: 19/20
Body composition: 5/20
OVERALL: 34/60

UP ESTROGEN CONTROL

WHAT? DIM/resveratrol/broccophane/green tea/turmeric/calcium-D-glucarate.

WHEN? 1–2 caps with breakfast.

WHY? We swim in a sea of estrogen in this modern world. This product contains proven nutraceuticals that assist the body in healthy estrogen management, leading to improved health, testosterone balance, and reduced female fat deposits such as 'man boobs'.

Health: 15/20
Performance: 4/20
Body composition: 14/20
OVERALL: 33/60

UP SLEEP ENHANCE

WHAT? L-theanine/phenibut/valerian extract.

WHEN? 1–2 caps at bedtime.

WHY? You do not need this supplement if you are able to fall asleep quickly and stay asleep for the duration of your time in bed. If your sleep is impaired, however, then this will limit your body composition results, and experimenting with supplements that help relax the nervous system and improve your circadian clock can be of significant benefit. Before buying any sleep-enhancing supplements please refer to the advice in Chapter 2 on how to improve your sleep.

Health: 10/20
Performance: 5/20
Body composition: 10/20
OVERALL: 25/60

UP TESTOSTERONE CONTROL

WHAT? Maca/tribulus/fenugreek.

WHEN? 2 caps twice daily, cycle on and off every two weeks.

WHY? Eliminate the idea that a supplement such as this can have a dramatic effect on your testosterone levels. In real terms it cannot, and the supplement company hype that promises 'steroid-like effects' is just shameless marketing lies. However, the right balance of herbs can temporarily improve the neurotransmitter dopamine, leading to improved focus, energy and sex drive.

Health: 4/20
Performance: 6/20
Body composition: 10/20
OVERALL: 20/60

WHEY PROTEIN

WHAT? A type of quickly absorbed protein derived from dairy products, typically found in powder form.

WHEN? 30–50g in a shake post-workout.

WHY? Whey protein is the king

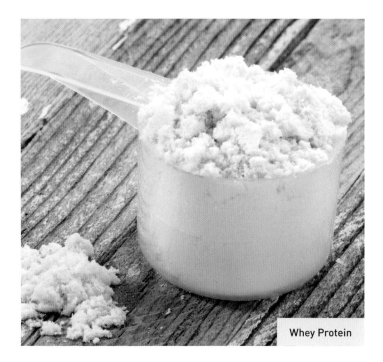

Whey Protein

ZINC

<u>WHAT?</u> Zinc is an essential mineral we can only get through our diet.
<u>WHEN?</u> 10mg per day.
<u>WHY?</u> We need zinc for hundreds of essential biological functions, not least for the production of testosterone, but many men have low levels. No one quite knows the reason why as yet but zinc appears, on a cellular level, to govern testosterone metabolism. This supplement restores adequate zinc levels for better muscle-building potential.

Health: 14/20
Performance: 5/20
Body composition: 12/20
<u>OVERALL: 31/60</u>

of all the protein powders. The reason for its importance is due to its extremely high score in something called the Biological Value scale. The BV scale is a measure of the quality of a specific protein source. The higher the score the more nitrogen your body would retain after eating it and the better it would help you stay anabolic (and, for our purposes, grow!).

Whey makes a great addition to your nutritional arsenal. As I have said in other parts of the book, never get so hooked on supplements that they replace food – this is a huge rookie error. However, whey post-workout is great because of its rapid absorption, and if you are caught short and unable to eat a solid meal then a whey shake plus a handful of nuts makes a great and healthy option.

Health: 10/20
Performance: 10/20
Body composition: 10/20
<u>OVERALL: 30/60</u>

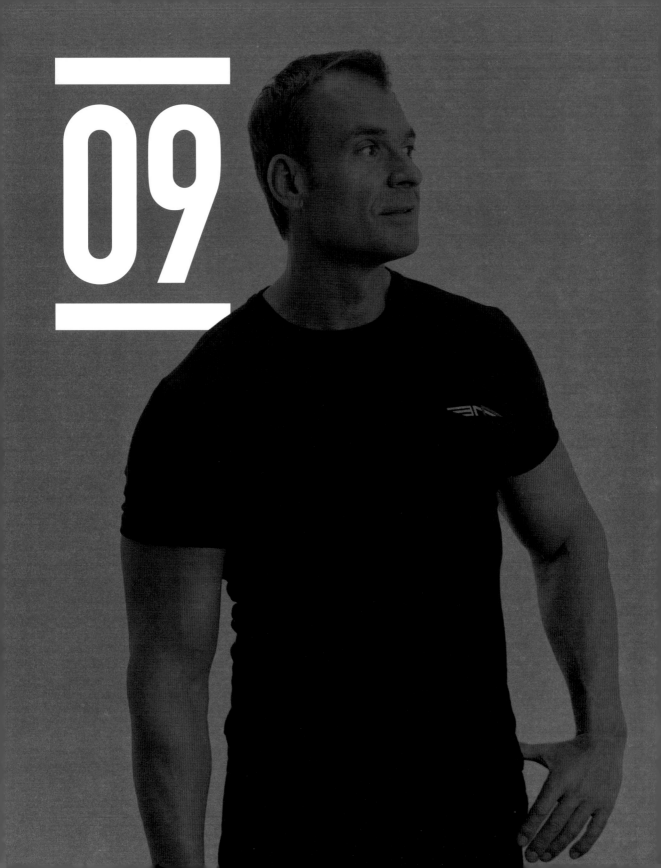

FREQUENTLY ASKED QUESTIONS

If you have a specific question for me then as long as it is about the programmes in this book, and you put the book cover as your profile picture when asking the question, I will answer you on Twitter (@HeyNickMitchell).

What's the deal with meal plans?

Let me make one thing abundantly clear to you. I hate meal plans!

I want you to think about this for a second: you probably can accept that you're a unique human being. You have unique goals, a unique tolerance for the boredom of a diet, and a truly unique set of daily circumstances that govern the how, the when and very often the 'what' of what goes into your mouth. And yet you expect me to be able to write you a meal plan that fits around all that?

What I want to do with my dietary advice is to give you an education, not prescriptive dogma. A meal plan doesn't allow you to deviate, to use common sense, or to adapt when things inevitably don't go exactly according to plan. If the meal plan says 'chicken and broccoli' and you've accidentally put in 'beef and carrots', what do you do? Sometimes it seems that 50 per cent of people panic and eat nothing, and the other 50 per cent think 'F*** it, let's eat chocolate.' Neither is the optimal choice.

Eating a healthy diet is pretty straightforward if you can stay focused enough to follow my basic rules. I know this is easier said than done because we are bombarded every day with marketing messages that 'low fat is best', 'cereals are healthy', and that something that is purple and you can squeeze out of a tube can count as part of our 'five a day'. Stick to my nutritional foundations and I promise you that it will be hard to go wrong and that you'll feel more energetic, sharper and leaner for the rest of your life.

Admittedly, things start to get a bit more complicated when we get into how to start to manipulate your diet for more aggressive fat loss and muscle building, but even then education and understanding are the key things to ensure your success.

And now I will proceed to completely contradict myself by referring you to Chapter 7 where you can find an extensive array of meal plans to suit all your transformation needs.

Why am I making such contradictory noises? Because experience has taught me that many people respond best to set rules over flexible choices. It's as simple as that.

Many of you won't need to use a meal plan as a guide, but some will find it mentally easier to just switch off and follow a fully laid-out plan. Neither option makes you a bad person. I care only about one thing: doing whatever it takes to help you achieve maximum results in minimum time.

Why did you list so many supplements?

We have listed a range of supplements covering a multitude of eventualities to give you a broader understanding of what is out there.

You are not expected or advised to take a plethora of supplements and you should note that during his 12-week programme our cover model only ever used a handful of products throughout the entire process.

I am on a tight budget. Shall I save up for supplements?

In a word – no. You should save your money for the best-quality food possible and forget about supplements. They are, by their very definition, 'supplementary' and come way behind spending money on the optimal training environment and good, real and wholesome food.

Can I substitute a shake for a meal?

In a perfect world you would be focusing on solid food for every meal other than the protein shake that you ingest immediately after a training session. However, many of you are busy, on the go, or struggle to chow down huge quantities of meat. I sympathise because this is an issue that I too struggle with.

Can we compromise and swap a meal for a shake? Yes we can, although we need to be aware of a few rules.

1. Other than post-workout try to have a whey shake with some sort of fibre: nuts if you are looking to keep calories higher, or some greens if getting lean is the primary aim. Of course,

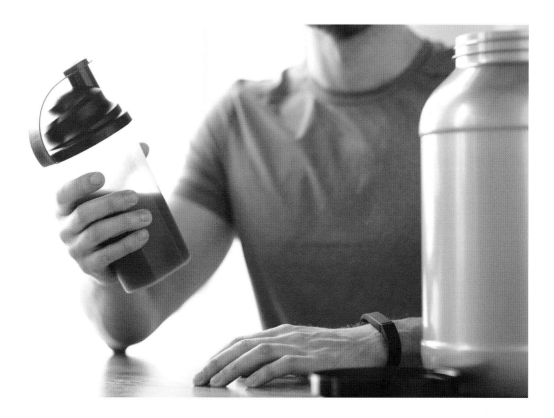

how many nuts and sundries you take is going to be down to your own specific diet so it's impossible to give you quantities. Even a very small handful can make a positive difference to your blood sugar.

2. I can accept one shake substitute a day (as well as your post-workout shake), but really try your best not to slip too far past that.

3. If you are struggling with eating your protein goal then finishing off a smaller meal with a protein shake that allows you to hit your protein goals is definitely a good idea.

Will my results be the same as Joe's?

Some people will do better than Joe and some won't quite achieve his heady heights of physical perfection. There are numerous reasons for this. The most obvious is that every single one of us is different – biochemically, hormonally, physiologically and mentally. I could take 1,000 members of the public and if I did exactly the same thing with each one of them (which, of course, I would never do) then we would have 1,000 different results.

Other factors that may mean your results differ from Joe's is that he had the advantage of training under me. Hopefully I am allowed to call myself a good coach, and what that means is that I know when to push hard, when to back off, and when to grind Joe through the floor. I also have my own gym so I can set things up perfectly. Both Joe and I know that the vast majority of you don't have that luxury and it is one of the reasons why we are giving as much information as possible in this book, and why we constantly make ourselves available via social media.

One of the things that I hear a lot is that person X follows programme Y 'perfectly' and doesn't get 'any' results. First of all, I have very rarely met someone who knows how to push as hard as possible in the gym, so that should always be the first thing to address. Second, so many of you cheat on your diets without ever realising it. This is where a food diary becomes supremely useful.

And finally, the expectations of results and reality can sometimes be ludicrously distorted. We have had people who spent 20 years getting overweight and who maybe have 50 pounds of fat to shift before they can ever see even an outline of abdominal muscle, complaining that there is no six-pack after a week.

Slow and steady wins the race with body-compositional improvements, and if you were to drop a very creditable 1.5lb of fat every week for 12 weeks you would be 18lb lighter and look and feel like a wholly different person.

What happens if I get injured?

If you are unfortunate enough to sustain an injury during the plan you have two choices – either crumble, undo all your hard work, and consume your bodyweight in junk food every day, or step up to the challenge, find a way to work around the injury, pay even more attention to your nutrition, and keep on improving, albeit at a reduced rate. The choice is yours, so don't BS yourself by self-indulgently thinking you can give up. Even being laid up in a hospital bed doesn't preclude you from eating properly.

As for how to treat an injury, I cannot give any specific information on that for obvious reasons. If you feel consulting a doctor would help then you must do that without hesitation, and if it is a niggle (or something more) that can be worked around then be sensible and avoid any movement at all that exacerbates the problem area.

As a little 'injury' bonus, my one piece of advice that I have seen help alleviate aches and pains more than anything else is the easiest and most straightforward for you to manage. Do everything that you can to minimise inflammation of your tissues, and the best way to do this is to eat a clean diet, with minimal sugar and junk food.

What will happen if I break my diet, and can I have a cheat meal?

Breaking your diet is not the end of the world and you should not let it signal a wholesale capitulation that sees you embark on a three-day bingeing frenzy. As soon as you break it, get back on the wagon and try to identify the triggers that caused you to stray in the first place so that you can avoid them next time.

One of the big problems that I see with people who are trying to radically alter their body composition is that too many are always asking 'When can I cheat?' This is the completely wrong mindset to have. Joe Warner didn't cheat once during his 12-week transformation, but he wanted to. In fact, at times he was a whining, moaning wreck craving certain foods. But he stayed strong because he had such a specific goal in mind and he had pushed the 'fear factor' onto himself of making his actions accountable to others (always a great lesson for getting a hard job done well).

I know that many of you have read about the concept of cheat meals 'stoking the metabolism'. This is true and not just some convenient urban dieter's myth. However, you need to be lean, mean and far into a strict diet before a cheat meal has any metabolic advantage. Of course, if a once-a-week modest cheat meal keeps you sane then by all means go for it, but stop kidding yourself that you 'need' it.

You can find many examples of how to use cheat meals and spike days at www.UltimateTransformation.Guide.

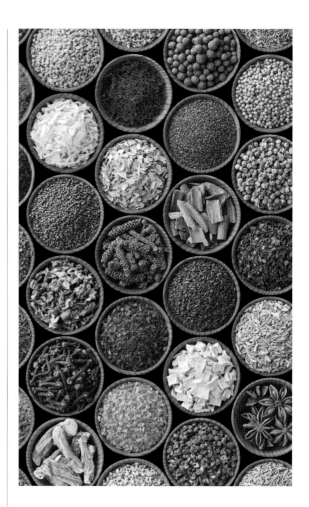

I can't stand bland foods!

You can spice foods to your heart's content. Just avoid too many excess calories, and sugary seasonings are best steered clear of altogether.

Many a bland diet has been saved with the liberal use of salt, garlic, onion, paprika, chilli, rosemary, thyme, vinegars, oregano, basil, cayenne pepper and cinnamon, to name but a few options.

Low carbs make me feel like a zombie!

Assuming you are sleeping correctly and not falling into the common pitfall of eating only protein (with both minimal fat and carbs) now is the time to start carb cycling.

I'm carb cycling for fat loss and progress has stalled!

The first thing to look at if you feel the plan isn't working is your food diary. What, you haven't been keeping one? This could be your first mistake. All too often we are surprised by what we eat when we keep a careful log. Some of you will be eating too much and some will be eating too little.

Assuming that you've been keeping a food diary and it looks OK, then we need to address training intensity. Have you been doing enough, and have you been training with sufficient intensity?

You also need to consider sleep and stress. Both are hugely influential factors in body composition progress.

If every box has been ticked off and carb cycling has still stalled then we have two obvious options. We go harder or we go easier. The harder option might mean dropping calories by a further 20 per cent for five days before returning to normal, and the easier option may be the entire opposite – increase calories by 20 per cent for five days before resuming your diet.

When my carbs go up what happens to protein and fat intake?

Carbohydrates are what we call 'protein sparing'. This means that your body will be far less likely to use protein for energy requirements if you are consuming sufficient carbohydrates, so on the days when we carb cycle higher we can knock down our protein intake a little bit. A good rule of thumb to start with is to take away 1g of protein for every 2g of extra carbs that you ingest, going no lower in protein intake than 1g per lb (not per kg!) of body weight per day.

We can also manipulate fat intake when carb cycling by going higher on (good) fats when lower in carbs and vice versa. My suggestion here is to keep an eye on your overall calorie intake and balance according to that. If you are adding an extra 400 calories of carbs, keeping protein the same (in this example), you may want to take out a certain number of calories from fat for that day. How much would really depend upon your goals and motivation.

I *must* count my calories. Is that OK?

It is now fashionable in certain circles to say that 'calories don't count'. In my opinion this is pure BS – if you eat 1,000 calories of nuts you might not get fat, but if you eat 10,000 calories of nuts then you will put on blubber. Case closed. However, counting calories can very often give a false impression of how you should eat, so for most of you I prefer to look at macronutrient intake, focusing much more on protein and carbs from the right sources (and letting fat take care of itself in many instances). To use a similar example to the above, do we think that 1,000 calories from chocolate will have the same physiological impact as 1,000 calories from beef and broccoli? I really hope that you don't think so.

My advice is to keep an eye on your calories and be aware that the leaner you become the more important manipulating them can be. But for 98 per cent of us focusing on macronutrient goals from our list of prescribed foods is the correct approach to adopt.

Can I substitute exercises?

There are three potential reasons why you may want and/or need to substitute an exercise from one of the programmes in this book:

- No access to the equipment: we have offered optional movements where certain less common equipment is needed.

- You feel injury pain when doing the exercise: this is the best excuse of all and you should never perform a movement that feels as though it is aggravating (in any way) an injury. Try to find the closest approximation that doesn't give you pain. For example, if your lower back feels dodgy doing barbell squats then try dumbbell squats or machine squats. You will need to think about this a little for yourself.

- The gym is too busy and you have no chance of getting on certain pieces of kit: again you must improvise and the best advice that I can give you without literally seeing your gym and taking you through a session is that we can mimic a heck of a lot of movements with just a pair of dumbbells.

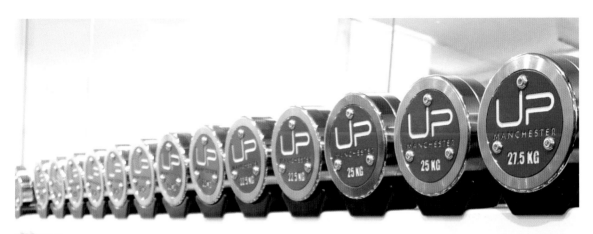

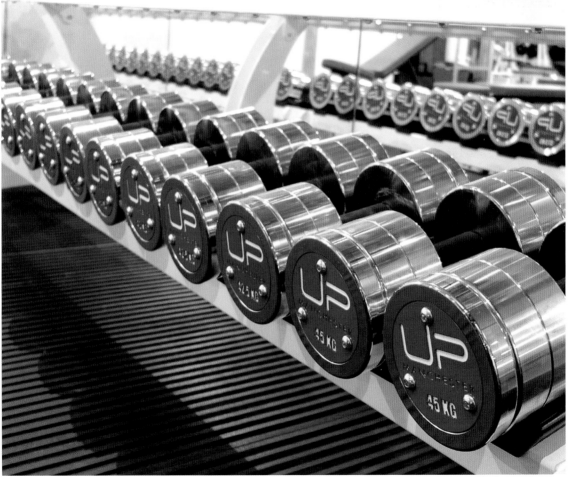

GLOSSARY

A quick guide to explain
some of the key terms
used in this book

Compound lift

This is a lift where movement occurs at two or more joints, such as a squat (movement at the hip and knee joints) or shoulder press (movement at the shoulder and elbow joints). Compound lifts should form the basis of all training programmes designed to increase muscle size, because they work more muscle groups at once.

Concentric contraction

A concentric contraction occurs when your muscle shortens to 'lift' the weight during each rep, such as the biceps shortening to raise a dumbbell from your side to shoulder-height during a biceps curl. Concentric contractions should be done fast but with control to work the muscle as forcefully as possible.

Eccentric contraction

An eccentric contraction occurs when your muscle lengthens to 'lower' the weight during each rep, such as the biceps lengthening to lower a dumbbell from your side to shoulder-height during a biceps curl. Eccentric contractions – also known as negative contractions – should be done slowly to work the muscle as thoroughly as possible. Your muscles are 10–20 per cent stronger during eccentric contractions than concentric contractions, which is why lowering a weight slowly and under control not only minimises the risk of injury, but also makes each rep more effective.

Isolation lift

This is a lift where movement occurs at one joint only, such as a biceps curl (movement at the elbow joint only) or leg extension (movement at the knee joint only). These moves are great for targeting a specific muscle group, especially at the end of a workout, to work the muscle really hard so it grows back bigger and stronger.

Isometric contraction

An isometric contraction occurs when a muscle generates force without changing length, such as during an abdominals plank, or when you grip an object using the muscles in your hand and wrist. These contractions don't typically generate as much force as either concentric or eccentric contractions, but they are still an important part of muscle growth.

Range of motion

This is the extent to which a joint or joints move during each rep. It is essential that you move through the fullest range of motion possible when performing a lift, because the greater the movement range, the more muscle fibres are recruited to move the weight, meaning you'll get a better muscle stretch and contraction with every rep.

Reps

An abbreviation of 'repetition'. One rep is the completion of a given exercise from the start position to the end position, moving through the full range of motion. The number of reps per set can vary depending on the training goal.

Rest

This is simply how long you rest between completing a set before starting the next one. If rest periods are too short then you will still be too fatigued to complete the following set; too long and you won't build up accumulated fatigue, which is essential for muscle-mass growth and burning body fat.

Sets

A set is a given number of reps performed consecutively without rest. The number of sets can vary for each exercise depending on the training goal.

Supersets

Supersets are two different exercises done back to back. Training this way is a proven method to promote muscle growth, because you can work more muscle groups in less time. Supersets are also a great way to encourage fat burning because you are forcing your heart and lungs to pump blood and oxygen to your muscles more quickly.

Tempo

Tempo is the speed at which you lift and lower a weight during each rep. The slower the tempo, the longer your muscles must work to manage and control the weight. This length of time is called time under tension. Tempo is detailed by a four-digit code, such as 2010. The first number is the time in seconds that the weight is lowered; the next number is the time in seconds that the move is held at the bottom position; the third number is the time in seconds that the weight is lifted; and the final digit is the time in seconds that the weight is held at the top of the move.

Time under tension

Time under tension is the duration in seconds that your muscles must work to control a weight during a single set, and it is dictated by the tempo multiplied by the count per set. For example, a set of 12 reps at a 2010 tempo (2 + 0 + 1 + 0 = 3 seconds) equals a total time under tension of 36 seconds for the set. Time under tension is one of the most important factors responsible for muscle-mass growth, which is why it is so important that you always stick to the tempo listed for each exercise, even if that means lowering the weight to achieve this.

LIST OF EXERCISES AND INDEX

LIST OF EXERCISES

INDEX

ACKNOWLEDGEMENTS

It's probably the goal of every lifelong gym rat to set all of his ideas down in one grand tome. I'd still be thinking about it rather than doing it if it weren't for the support and confidence of my wonderful family, friends and colleagues.

First and foremost, everything that I do is made possible because I am supported at home by Marcela Kubinova. I'm the quarterback who gets to make the flashy pass, and endure the odd sack, but she is the one who gets me safely onto the field of play every time. Without her unflinching devotion I could never have had the opportunity to have my cake and eat it, working on my career and enjoying the beautiful family that she looks after with a heart of gold and a rod of Slavic iron.

My children, Roman and Mia, are my inspirations. Roman was also Joe Warner's inspiration when the six-year-old beat the thirty-three-year-old in a sprint race at the start of Joe's 12-week transformation!

In a way I need an entire chapter to thank my two-time cover model and collaborator Joe Warner, but I'll have to opt for brevity. He threw himself into the 12-week process with full commitment, and despite his own ridiculously busy schedule as the editor and publisher of two magazines, *Iron Life* and *Alpha Man*, he was prepared to uproot his life and come and live on my home turf in Marbella for three months. His honesty, his professionalism and his friendship were all instrumental factors in enabling me to devote the time it takes to prepare a book like this. It's trite to write 'I couldn't have done it without him,' but nothing could be closer to the truth.

The ideas in this book are the product of thirty years of experience. I've not learned these things by being stuck in a dungeon, and I have benefited from the help of more people than I could possibly mention. I learned what real training was all about at Muscleworks Gym in London, and I'll forever owe a debt of gratitude to Savvas Kyriacou and all the great bodybuilders who came up there in the 1990s. Louis Durkin was always the perfect in-the-gym trainer when he wanted to be, and a part of the results that the dedicated reader will get from this book are down to the ideas that he sparked in my mind.

The training routines in this book have Charles Poliquin's influence stamped all over them. No one teaches better programming than Charles, and I am proud to call him my friend. He has always been there for me to tell me if he thinks one of my ideas is great or 'dweebish'. Just as it should be; there's never any beating around the bush.

There'd be no book if my great friend Mike Weeks had not introduced me to the great agent Robert Kirby. Thank you both for helping to get the show on the road. And thanks to the HarperCollins team: Carolyn Thorne, Orlando Mowbray, Simon Gerratt, Sim Greenaway, James Empringham and Dean Russell.

The laboratory where I've really tested all my ideas has been the Ultimate Performance (UP) gym floor. An enormous amount of credit for my ability to write this book goes to everyone in our worldwide team. There are one hundred plus of you to thank as a collective, but individually Joe Halstead, whom I trust like a brother and who steers me with his analysis; Glenn Parker, who has been at UP from before there even was UP; Eddie Baruta, who can always be counted on when the chips are down; Akash Vaghela, for his detailed work on the meal plans; and Ridhi Sharma, who is always there for me when I need her.

And I couldn't have even made it to the starting line without Anne and Michael Mitchell, my parents. They gave me the confidence to believe that as long as I was prepared to work harder than anyone else then I could do anything at all I wanted to do with my life. In a way that is the key message I want the reader to take from this book.